MW01676435

The Appropriateness of Manipulation and Mobilization of the Cervical Spine

Ian D. Coulter, Eric L. Hurwitz, Alan H. Adams,
William C. Meeker, Dan T. Hansen, Robert D. Mootz,
Peter D. Aker, Barbara J. Genovese, Paul G. Shekelle

Supported by the
Consortium for Chiropractic Research

RAND

PREFACE

This report presents results from the RAND study on the appropriateness of spinal manipulation and mobilization of the cervical spine. The study was designed to ascertain the clinical criteria for the appropriate use of cervical manipulation and mobilization to treat conditions such as neck pain and headache and to document treatment complications.

An extensive review of the medical and chiropractic literature was conducted to summarize knowledge about efficacy, complications, and indications for manipulation and mobilization of the cervical spine. From this literature of 507 articles, a set of indications was created for manipulation and mobilization for neck pain and headaches and for subcategories of patient types. A panel was convened of experts from the disciplines of orthopedics, chiropractic, family medicine, neurosurgery, and neurology to rate for appropriateness the indications for spinal manipulation and mobilization.

The set of indications derived from the literature and informed sources was circulated to the panel and rated individually by each panelist for appropriateness for manipulation and mobilization. The panel of experts was convened to rate the same indications for mobilization and manipulation of the cervical spine following reporting and discussion of the previous ratings.

This report presents the results of the final ratings. It describes the methods used for assessing and rating the appropriateness of 1,436 indications for the use of spinal manipulation and mobilization of the cervical spine. These findings should be of interest to clinicians (particularly in the disciplines of chiropractic, physical therapy, osteopathy, and physical medicine) who perform manipulation and mobilization of the cervical spine, to clinicians who deal with patients with cervical problems, and to health researchers concerned with the appropriate indications for performing manipulation and mobilization.

This research is a joint undertaking of the Consortium for Chiropractic Research, the Los Angeles College of Chiropractic; the Palmer College of Chiropractic, West; and RAND.

CONTENTS

FIGURES

TABLES

SUMMARY

INTRODUCTION

This report contains a literature review of 507 articles and the indications and ratings for appropriateness of spinal manipulation and mobilization of the cervical spine that reflect the findings of a nine-member multidisciplinary panel comprised of four chiropractors, four medical physicians, and one individual who is both a chiropractor and a medical physician. The panel members rated the appropriateness of indications twice, using a nine-point scale where 1 = extremely inappropriate, 5 = uncertain, and 9 = extremely appropriate. The panelists were chosen because of their clinical expertise, professional repute, and diversity of geographic location. Furthermore, they represent both academic and community practice.

LITERATURE REVIEW

Spinal manipulation and mobilization are used as a treatment modality for an array of conditions, including back pain, neck pain, headache, and other somatic and non-somatic conditions. The purpose of this review is to assess the evidence for the use of cervical spine manipulation for the treatment of a range of conditions, primarily neck pain and headache, and to document the complications resulting from its use. Spinal manipulation, for the purpose of this review, is a controlled, judiciously applied dynamic thrust (adjustment) that may include combined extension and rotation of the upper cervical spinal segments, or low-velocity and low-amplitude force with the use of a short or long lever directed to spinal joint segments within patient tolerance. These procedures often take joints into the "paraphysiological" space resulting in joint cavitation. Clinical trials of treatments employing mobilization techniques are also included in this review. Mobilization is defined as a controlled, judiciously applied force of low velocity and variable amplitude directed to spinal joint segment(s). A typical contact position for cervical manipulation is shown in Figure 1.

Structured database searching and consultation with experts were used to identify studies which after further review for relevance yielded 362 primary articles on cervical spine manual therapy and 145 articles on complications resulting from such therapy.

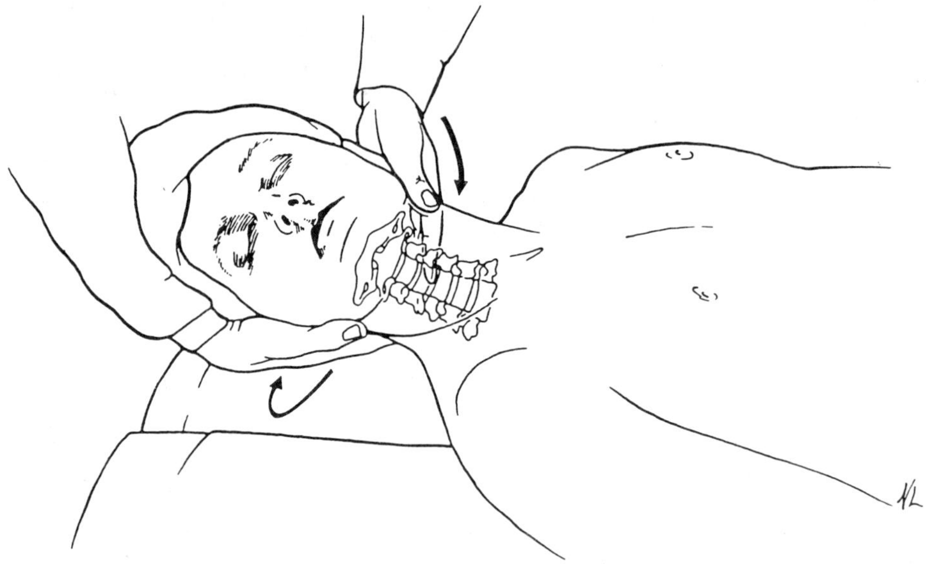

Figure 1—Schematic Representation of an Upper Cervical Adjustment[1]

Focus and Criteria

First priority was given to research that used a randomized, controlled trial (RCT) design. Second priority was given to nonexperimental studies, including cohort, case-control, and cross-sectional studies. Case series and case reports were given lowest priority and were included only for completeness and to document the use of cervical manipulation for conditions for which there was little or no other evidence available. This process generated 108 studies or reports that were judged to deal with efficacy, from the total 362 articles: 16 RCTs, 13 cohort studies, 27 case series, and 52 case reports. The review includes data from the 108 studies. The criteria used for assessing the studies of efficacy were taken from Koes et al. (1991).

Neck pain. Five RCTs, one cohort study, four case series, and 24 case reports were identified that attempted to assess the effectiveness of cervical spine manipulation for the treatment of neck pain. An additional four RCTs, one cohort study, and one case series dealt with, at least in part, the effectiveness of mobilization for neck pain. The manipulation RCTs focused primarily on subacute and chronic neck pain, whereas four of the mobilization RCTs addressed acute neck pain.

Acute neck pain. No RCTs or case series were found that present data about the efficacy of cervical spine manipulation specifically for patients with acute neck pain. The limited literature available on mobilization for acute neck pain indicates that it may be beneficial for some patients, at least compared to rest and cervical collar, although instruction on mobilization and exercises may be equally beneficial.

---

[1]The original line drawing appears in T. Bergman, D. Peterson, and D. Lawrence, *Chiropractic Technique,* New York: Churchill Livingstone, 1993, and is used with the publisher's permission.

Subacute and chronic neck pain. Five RCTs of manipulation and one RCT of mobilization for subacute or chronic neck pain were reviewed. Seven other studies provided additional data. Evidence from the literature reveals that cervical spine manipulation and/or mobilization may provide at least short-term pain relief and range of motion enhancement for persons with subacute or chronic neck pain. The published results are insufficient to make efficacy determinations separately for patients with subacute pain and patients with chronic neck pain.

Headache. Five RCTs, 10 case series, and 19 case reports were identified that assess the effectiveness of cervical spine manipulation for headache. One additional RCT addressed, in part, the effectiveness of mobilization techniques for headache.

Muscle tension headache. Four RCTs of manipulation and one RCT of mobilization for headache were reviewed. Nine other studies provided additional data. The literature is sparse but suggests that cervical spine manipulation and/or mobilization may provide short-term relief for some patients with muscle tension (and other nonmigraine) headaches. The evidence for long-term benefit is much less conclusive.

Migraine headache. One RCT and five other studies of manipulation for migraine headache were reviewed. The literature is too limited to support or to refute the use of cervical spine manipulation and/or mobilization for patients suffering from migraine headaches.

Shoulder/arm/hand pain. *Acute, subacute, and chronic pain.* The literature, consisting of data from a single RCT and two case series, is insufficient to support or to refute the use of cervical spine manipulation and/or mobilization for patients with pain of any duration of the shoulder, arm, and/or hand.

Thoracic Outlet Syndrome, Carpal Tunnel Syndrome, TMJ disorders. No RCTs were found to support manipulation or mobilization for any of these conditions. Isolated case reports record clinical improvement in some patients.

Blood pressure and heart rate, cervical spine/intersegmental motion, cervical spine curvature, miscellaneous conditions. Insufficient evidence exists to support or to refute the use of cervical spine mobilization or manipulation for most of the above entities. However, the literature does provide evidence that manipulation of the cervical spine increases range of motion and intersegmental mobility. The clinical significance of this finding is not known.

Complications

Articles documenting more than 110 cases of complications allegedly arising from cervical spine manipulation have been published in English. The vast majority of these complications involved vertebrobasilar accidents (VBA) with consequences such as brainstem and/or cerebellar infarction, Wallenberg's Syndrome (obstruction of the posterior inferior cerebellar artery), and Locked-in Syndrome (occlusion of basilar artery). Other reported complications include spinal cord compression, vertebral fracture, tracheal rupture, diaphragm paralysis, internal carotid hematoma, and cardiac arrest.

Frequency of Complications

It is difficult to estimate the frequency of vertebrobasilar accidents and other complications among patients undergoing cervical spine manipulation because of the uncertainty of both caseload and the number of cervical manipulations that patients receive over a given period of time. The risk of complications has been estimated to be between one in 40,000 manipulations for mild complications and one in 400,000 to more than one million manipulations for serious complications. No serious neurological complications were found during one year among 460 physicians and approximately 150,000 cervical manipulations in one large case series.

Based on the best available evidence, we estimate the rate of complications as a result of cervical spine manipulation to be one per one million manipulations.

RATINGS

The literature review, a set of clinical indications, and instructions for making ratings of appropriateness were mailed to the panelists. The initial ratings of appropriateness were done individually, without group discussion. The second-round ratings used a structured method, which was based on consensus procedures developed for the RAND/UCLA Health Services Utilization Study.[1]

The results showed that these physicians were able to formulate detailed lists of indications for cervical manipulation and to rate the appropriateness of each.

An increase in agreement and a decrease in disagreement arose between the initial round and the second round. The final round rated 1,436 indications, with disagreement on 2 percent of the indications. The final round rated 43 percent of the indications as inappropriate for manipulation or mobilization. Appropriate and uncertain indications each accounted for 41 percent and 16 percent of the total, respectively. The frequency with which indications occur in a population of patients is unknown and will require additional data collection to determine the rate of appropriate use of cervical spine manipulation and mobilization.

---

[1]A complete discussion of this method is given in R. H. Brook, "Appropriateness Method," *Clinical Practice Guideline Development: Methodologic Perspectives*, Rockville, Md.: AHCPR, Public Health Services, 1993.

ACKNOWLEDGMENTS

The authors are indebted to the nine members of the spinal manipulation panel:

Arthur Croft, D.C.
Coronado, Calif.

Peter Curtis, M.D.
University of North Carolina
Department of Family Medicine
Chapel Hill, N.C.

Thomas B. Ducker, M.D.
Annapolis, Md.

Ronald Evans, D.C.
Des Moines, Ia.

Steve Garfin, M.D.
University of California, San Diego
Medical Center
San Diego, Calif.

George McClelland, D.C.
Christianburg, Va.

David Sherman, M.D.
Department of Medicine
University of Texas Health Sciences Center
San Antonio, Tex.

Rand Swenson, M.D., Ph.D., D.C.
Monadnock Hospital
Peterborough, N.H.

Howard Vernon, D.C.
Canadian Memorial Chiropractic College
Toronto, Ontario, Canada.

Chapter One

METHODS

The indications and ratings for spinal manipulation for neck pain and headache reported here reflect the findings of a nine-member panel of clinicians who rated indications twice. The initial ratings of appropriateness were made individually, without group discussion. The second-round ratings followed a structured method based on procedures often used to bring people closer to consensus or agreement. These ratings were conducted using the method developed during the RAND/UCLA Health Services Utilization Study and described in detail elsewhere.[1]

The panelists were chosen on the basis of their clinical expertise, professional repute (in professional organizations, for example), and diversity of geographic location, with all four major census regions and Canada represented. Also, the panelists were selected to represent a combination of academic and community practice.

The panel was chosen from individuals nominated by influential, opinion leaders in the field of cervical care. From the medical profession, nominations were sought in the areas of orthopedics, neurosurgery, neurology, and primary care. The final list of individuals was then reviewed by other opinion leaders. For the chiropractic members, recommendations were sought from both the Consortium for Chiropractic Research and the Foundation for Chiropractic Education and Research. Again, the final list was reviewed by opinion leaders.

PANELISTS:

Dr. Arthur Croft, a chiropractor in general practice who has published widely on whiplash and cervical injuries.

Dr. Peter Curtis, an academic primary care physician trained in physical manipulation.

Dr. Thomas Ducker, an academic neurosurgeon and editor of a major professional journal on the spine.

Dr. Ronald Evans, a chiropractor in general practice.

[1]A complete discussion of this method is given in R. H. Brook, "Appropriateness Method," *Clinical Practice Guideline Development: Methodologic Perspectives,* Rockville, Md.: AHCPR, Public Health Service, 1993.

Dr. Steve Garfin, an academic orthopedic surgeon and associate editor of a major professional journal dealing with the spine.

Dr. George McClelland, a chiropractor in general practice.

Dr. David Sherman, an academic neurologist who has published in the area of complications of cervical spine manipulation.

Dr. Rand Swenson, an academic neurologist with a doctorate in anatomy, who also trained as a chiropractor.

Dr. Howard Vernon, an academic chiropractor who has conducted research and published in the area of headache.

INITIAL INDICATIONS LIST

The project staff compiled the initial indications list using the literature review and the advice of chiropractors, medical physicians, and physical therapists. The indications categorized persons in terms of their history, symptoms, physical and radiographic findings, and response to prior treatment. We attempted to compile lists that were detailed, comprehensive, and manageable. The lists needed enough detail so that patients presenting with a particular indication would be relatively homogeneous, in the sense that doing the procedure would be equally appropriate (or inappropriate) for all of them. We sought to include all indications for doing cervical manipulation or mobilization that might arise in practice. At the same time, we tried to keep the total number of indications low enough to allow the panelists to rate all of them within a reasonable length of time.

Using the initial indications list, a group of chiropractic consultants developed a structure designed to reflect both the literature review, which was provided to them, and their clinical experience. This list and structure were then reviewed and modified by a general internist in consultation with project staff and medical experts staff to ensure completeness, specificity, and comprehensiveness and to incorporate clinical logic comprehensible to allopathic physicians.

Our initial list of indications was modified by the multidisciplinary expert panel to better fit their clinical experience. We used this final indications list as the framework for the appropriateness ratings by the expert panel in round two.

The indications were organized into 13 "chapters" which clustered indications within major symptoms or primary problems. The chapter titles f are as follows:

1. Acute neck pain and signs of painful and/or limited active range of motion and pain anatomically consistent with a musculotendinous distribution and no radiculopathy.
2. Subacute or chronic neck pain and signs of painful and/or limited active range of motion and pain anatomically consistent with a musculotendinous distribution and no radiculopathy.

3. Peripheral pain of probable sclerotogenous distribution.
4. Pain consistent with musculotendinous involvement of the temporomandibular joint (TMJ).
5. Acute neck pain and clinical suspicion of cervical nerve root involvement.
6. Subacute or chronic neck pain and clinical suspicion of cervical nerve root involvement.
7. Generalized neck pain.
8. Acute constant headache.
9. Acute or subacute intermittent headache.
10. Chronic intermittent headache.
11. Persistent neuralgic pain consistent with cranial nerve distribution; insidious facial palsy; idiopathic insidious vertigo and/or dizziness; insidious spasmodic torticollis in the absence of congenital, postsurgical, or postfracture etiologies; or idiopathic insidious pharyngeal dysfunction.
12. Miscellaneous (with radiographic evidence).
13. Miscellaneous (cardiovascular related conditions).

INITIAL RATINGS

The panel members were sent the literature review included in this report, along with ratings sheets and a set of instructions. The literature review gave all panelists equal access to a central core of relevant literature. The rating sheets listed 1,171 indications for manipulation and mobilization and provided space for an appropriateness rating on a scale of 1 to 9. Figure 2 contains the instructions given to the panel.

The instructions asked the panelists to use their own best clinical judgment considering an average group of patients presenting to an average provider who performed manipulation and mobilization. Although "average provider" is not predefined for the panel members in the RAND consensus panels, it is discussed in the panel so that there is a common understanding. In general terms, an average provider is neither the best nor the worst provider. The RAND consensus method is designed to look at the appropriateness by an average provider trained in that procedure. In the case of manipulation, this would include chiropractors, osteopaths, physical therapists, and physicians in manual medicine. The present panelists are familiar with these providers and their level of competence. The RAND method is not designed to explicitly address the issue of who is the most competent provider. The method assumes the therapy is competently delivered, and the ratings reflect this assumption. Appropriate care was defined to mean that expected health benefits to the patient (e.g., increase life expectancy, relief of symptoms, reduction of

*1. **Format of the Indications***

The rating forms are organized in 13 chapters by clinical presentation. Within each chapter you will be asked to rate the appropriateness of performing cervical spinal manipulation or mobilization for different, clinically specific indications for the procedure.

See the sample rating page included. The clinical presentation is patients who present with neck pain with painful or limited range of motion and no radiculopathy. Thirty-six nine-point scales are shown. Each scale represents one of the 36 possible combinations of critical factors. The first combination of critical factors listed under heading "A" represents a patient with a non-traumatic or minimally traumatic etiology of their pain, who has had no cervical spine radiographs performed and who does not have clinical risk factors for contraindications for cervical manipulation, and who has never before been treated with spinal manipulative therapy. A list of definitions of subjective terms can be found following this set of instructions.

*2. **The Appropriateness Rating Scale***

You are asked to rate the clinical appropriateness of performing cervical spinal manipulation or mobilization using a nine-point scale as follows:

Appropriateness Ratings	Relationship of Benefits to Risks
1	Risks greatly exceed benefits
2	—
3	—
4	—
5	Benefits and risks about equal
6	—
7	—
8	—
9	Benefits greatly exceed risks

For 1994, please tell us how appropriate it is to perform cervical spinal manipulation or mobilization for each specified clinical indication. You are free to use any of the nine points on the scale to define the degree of appropriateness you feel pertains to each definition.

By "appropriate" we mean that expected health benefits to the patient (e.g., increase life expectancy, relief of symptoms, reduction of anxiety, improved functional capacity, etc.) exceed expected health risks (e.g., mortality, morbidity, pain produced by the procedure) by a sufficiently wide margin that the procedure is worth doing.

You should evaluate benefits and risks based on commonly accepted best clinical practice for the year 1994. Consider an average group of patients with each listed indication, presenting to an average practitioner in the United States who performs spinal manipulation. The ratings should reflect your own best clinical judgment.

Figure 2—Instructions to Panel for Reviewing and Rating Indications for Cervical Spine Manipulation and Mobilization.

anxiety, improved functional capacity) exceeded expected health risks (e.g., mortality, morbidity, pain produced by the procedure) by a sufficiently wide margin that the procedure is worth doing. Extremely appropriate indications should be rated 9, extremely inappropriate 1, and indications for which the risks and benefits were about equal (or unknown) were to be rated a 5. The instructions also included definitions of important terms. Furthermore, the panelists were encouraged to modify and supplement the indications lists to make them more complete and more clinically relevant, but few changes were recommended prior to the meeting of the panel.

PANEL MEETINGS

The cervical manipulation panel met in Santa Monica, California, for one day on June 17, 1994. The panelists spent the entire day discussing and re-rating the indications.

The discussion was jointly chaired by a medical physician and a chiropractic physician who participated in creating the indications list, were familiar with the literature, and were experienced in the consensus process. They were assisted by other project staff.

After discussing and agreeing on the definitions (see Appendix A), the panelists discussed and re-rated each chapter. During these discussions, each panelist had individual copies of reports that summarized the initial ratings for that chapter. Figure 3 shows one page of the report for one panelist.

From the printout of the ratings from the first round, each panelist could see the distribution of the responses of the initial ratings (the scales of 1 to 9 in Figure 3) and how many panelists assigned each rating. In addition, each panelist saw his or her own rating. However, no panelist was shown the individual ratings of another panelist, and, therefore, each panelist received a different rating report. The distribution of the ratings is the same on all reports, but the caret (^) below the rating line indicates the panelist's own rating. This procedure preserved the confidentiality of individual ratings but gave the distribution of ratings for the entire group and the individual's own rating for that indication.

The indications list from round 1 was revised during the discussion (the number of indications increased from 1,171 to 1,436). The changes were intended to make the indications better fit clinically relevant categories and to make the groups more homogeneous with respect to appropriateness. For example "psychosocial stress" became "significant psychosocial stress" and "depression" became "diagnosed depression."

```
panelist 1;  round 1;  page  2                                                       Fri Nov 17 14:46:54 1995
-----------------------------------------------------------------------------------------------------------------
Chapter 2
CERVICAL SPINAL MANIPULATION OR MOBILIZATION
IS APPROPRIATE WITH:
SUBACUTE OR CHRONIC NECK PAIN AND SIGNS OF
PAINFUL AND/OR LIMITED ACTIVE RANGE OF MOTION   NO OTHER ADEQUATE CONSERVATIVE      NONMANIPULATIVE CONSERVATIVE CARE
AND PAIN ANATOMICALLY CONSISTENT WITH A            CARE FOR THIS EPISODE             FOR THIS EPISODE HAS FAILED
MUSCULOTENDINOUS DISTRIBUTION AND              ------------------------------------  ------------------------------------
NO RADICULOPATHY AND                            Mobilization        Manipulation      Mobilization        Manipulation
-----------------------------------------------------------------------------------------------------------------
CONTINUED BIOMECHANICAL OR PSYCHOSOCIAL
STRESS AND

A. Non-traumatic or minimally traumatic
   etiology and no prior experience with SMT
   AND

   1. No cervical spine radiographs and
      absence of clinical risk factors for
      contraindications for cervical                 1   1 1 2 4    2       1 1 4 1        1       4 4    1 1       1 4 2
      manipulation                                 1 2 3 4 5 6 7 8 9  1 2 3 4 5 6 7 8 9  1 2 3 4 5 6 7 8 9  1 2 3 4 5 6 7 8 9      (  1-  4)
                                                             ^                  ^                    ^                    ^
   2. No cervical spine radiographs and
      presence of clinical risk factors for
      contraindications for cervical               1 1   1 2 1 3      2 2 2   3          1 1 1     3 2 1    2 3     2 2
      manipulation                                 1 2 3 4 5 6 7 8 9  1 2 3 4 5 6 7 8 9  1 2 3 4 5 6 7 8 9  1 2 3 4 5 6 7 8 9      (  5-  8)
                                                           ^                  ^                    ^                  ^
   3. Absence of clinical and radiographic
      risk factors for contraindications for                   3 4 2          2   2 3 2              2 4 3          2   1 2 4
      cervical manipulation                        1 2 3 4 5 6 7 8 9  1 2 3 4 5 6 7 8 9  1 2 3 4 5 6 7 8 9  1 2 3 4 5 6 7 8 9      (  9- 12)
                                                                 ^                    ^                ^                    ^
B. Non-traumatic or minimally traumatic
   etiology and favorable prior experience
   with SMT AND

   1. No cervical spine radiographs and
      absence of clinical risk factors for
      contraindications for cervical                       1 2 2 3 1    1   1   1 2 3 1            2 2 4 1    1   1     1 5 1
      manipulation                                 1 2 3 4 5 6 7 8 9  1 2 3 4 5 6 7 8 9  1 2 3 4 5 6 7 8 9  1 2 3 4 5 6 7 8 9      ( 13- 16)
                                                             ^                    ^                  ^                    ^
   2. No cervical spine radiographs and
      presence of clinical risk factors for
      contraindications for cervical               1     2 1 2 3      1 2 2   3 1              1 1 3 1 2    1 2 1 1 1 1 1
      manipulation                                 1 2 3 4 5 6 7 8 9  1 2 3 4 5 6 7 8 9  1 2 3 4 5 6 7 8 9  1 2 3 4 5 6 7 8 9      ( 17- 20)
                                                           ^                    ^                  ^                    ^
   3. Absence of clinical and radiographic
      risk factors for contraindications for                   4 3 2        1     1 1 3 3              3 2 4        1   1     2 5
      cervical manipulation                        1 2 3 4 5 6 7 8 9  1 2 3 4 5 6 7 8 9  1 2 3 4 5 6 7 8 9  1 2 3 4 5 6 7 8 9      ( 21- 24)
                                                                 ^                    ^                ^                    ^
-----------------------------------------------------------------------------------------------------------------
Appropriateness scale:  1 = extremely inappropriate,   5 = uncertain,   9 = extremely appropriate.
```

Figure 3—Example of a Panel Rating Form

Chapter Two

LITERATURE REVIEW OF MANIPULATION AND MOBILIZATION OF THE CERVICAL SPINE

INTRODUCTION

Spinal manipulation is used as a treatment modality for an array of conditions, including back pain, neck pain, headache, and other somatic and nonsomatic conditions. Recently, research has focused on the efficacy of spinal manipulation for the treatment of low-back pain (Shekelle et al., 1992). The purpose of this review is to assess the evidence for the use of cervical spine manipulation for the treatment of a range of conditions, primarily neck pain and headache, and to document the complications resulting from its use. Spinal manipulation, for the purpose of this review, is a controlled judiciously applied dynamic thrust (adjustment) that may include combined extension and rotation of the upper cervical spinal segments or low-velocity and low-amplitude force with the use of a short or long lever directed to spinal joint segments within patient tolerance. Studies employing mobilization techniques are also included in this review. Mobilization includes any manual therapy directed at joint dysfunction that does not involve a high-velocity thrust. Studies describing manipulation with instrumentation (e.g., activator), manipulation under anesthesia (MUA), or manual therapies that are not directed at influencing joint function (e.g., traction) are excluded.

METHODS

A structured database search of four computerized bibliographic databases (MEDLINE [*Index Medicus*], EMBASE [*Exerpta Medica*], CHIROLARS [*Chiropractic*], and CINAHL [*Cumulative Index of Nursing and Allied Health Literature*]) was performed to identify English-only citations from 1966 to the present. Databases with start dates after 1966 were searched from the earliest possible time. Searching of these four databases allowed for the retrieval of citations from allopathic medicine in North America and Europe, manual medicine, chiropractic, osteopathic, physiotherapy, nursing, and dental temporomandibular joint (TMJ) literature.

The literature search targeted information on the efficacy of cervical spine manipulation. The retrieval incorporated anatomical (cervical spine) and therapeutic (manipulation) terms and also broad disorder terms such as neck pain, headache, and whiplash, as well as TMJ disorders, face pain, cervical angina, and other simulated visceral conditions. Keywords and search strategies were selected in cooperation with an expert librarian with previous experience in computerized health literature database searches.

Our search strategy identified 1,457 citations, which were reviewed for first-round relevancy criteria by one investigator (a chiropractor). These criteria allowed inclusion of all citations relating to manual therapy of the cervical spine. As a result of this first-round relevancy screening, 705 citations were identified as relevant: 560 on cervical spine manual therapies and 145 on complications from manual therapy to the cervical spine. These citations were then retrieved and reviewed with stricter relevancy criteria by two investigators (both chiropractors). These second-round relevancy criteria allowed inclusion of all articles on utilization, efficacy, and complications of cervical spine manipulation and excluded those on technique descriptions, diagnostic tests, outcome reliability, or other material that did not use or describe manual therapy of the cervical spine as an intervention.

Upon completion of this screening process, 362 primary articles on cervical spine manual therapy and 145 articles on complications were identified. Two additional randomized controlled trials (one published and one submitted) on cervical spine manipulation were available from the personal files of one of the investigators. In all, 108 articles on efficacy included primary data. Finally, articles describing studies or case reports that did not employ high-velocity thrusts or mobilization techniques as part of the treatment protocol were excluded. Table 1 classifies studies that were used to assess the efficacy of cervical spine manipulation. Table 2 characterizes the complications from cervical spine manipulation. The latter are mainly case studies.

The randomized controlled trials (RCTs) were assessed for quality by two independent investigators using the scoring system of Koes and colleagues (Koes et al., 1991). The criteria used in the assessment are given in Table 1. This system was developed to assess the quality of RCTs of musculoskeletal therapies. This scoring system assigns points for the homogeneity, comparability, and follow-up of the study population; the descriptions of the interventions given; the types of outcome measures used and how they were assessed; and the data presentation and analysis. The maximum score is 100. These quality ratings were then reviewed by a third researcher. If disagreements between the two initial raters occurred, they were resolved by the ratings of the third rater and by consensus following discussion. The initial agreement between the two raters was in excess of 85 percent. In the final ratings, complete consensus was obtained.[1] When completed, the literature was further reviewed by a physician-methodologist (a person not otherwise associated with the project, i.e., external to the RAND peer reviewers), an orthopedist, and a physical therapist who practices cervical spine manipulation and lectures frequently on the topic.

---

[1]Although this method of rating studies has been extensively used, inter-rater reliability is not extensively reported in the literature. Since all disagreements are resolved consensually or by using a third blinded reviewer, the final agreement is 100 percent. Koes et al. (1991), in a recent study, report disagreement on 19 percent of 1,440 instances in which a criterion was applied. These disagreements were mostly a result of errors in reading, and were reduced to 4 after a consensus meeting involving a third reviewer. In a second study report, van der Wendt et al. (1995) achieved a 90 percent agreement for two initial raters. Detsky et al. (1992), in testing the Chalmers rating method and using four pairs of raters, obtained Spearman correlation coefficients ranging from 0.88 to 0.96 and an interclass correlation of 0.92 [(95 percent confidence level (CI), of 0.81–0.98)].

Table 1

Criteria for Assessing the Methods of Studies of Efficacy of Spinal Manipulation (Koes et al., 1991)

A	Description of inclusion and exclusion criteria (1 point). Restriction to a homogenous study population (1 point).
B	Comparability for duration of complaints, value of outcome measures, age, recurrences, and radiating complaints (1 point each).
C	Randomization procedure described (2 points). Randomization procedure that excludes bias (for example, sealed envelopes) (2 points).
D	Information about which group from which patients withdrew and reason for withdrawal (3 points).
E	Loss to follow-up: all randomized patients minus the number of patients at main point of measurement of the main outcome measure, divided by all randomized patients, multiplied by 100 (maximum, 4 points).
F	Smallest group immediately after randomization (> 50 subjects in smallest group, 6 points; > 100 subjects in smallest group, 6 additional points).
G	Manipulative treatment explicitly described (5 points). All reference treatments explicitly described (5 points).
H	Comparison with an established treatment (5 points).
I	Other physical treatments or medical interventions avoided in the design of the study (except analgesics; advice on posture; or use at home of heat, rest, or a routine exercise scheme) (5 points).
J	Comparison with placebo (5 points).
K	Citation of qualified education or experience, or both, of the manipulative therapist (5 points).
L	Placebo-controlled study: attempt at blinding (3 points), blinding evaluated and fully successful (2 points). Pragmatic study: patients fully naive (3 points) or time restriction (no manipulative treatment for at least 1 year) (2 points); naiveness evaluated and fully successful (2 points).
M	Measured and reported use of pain, global measurement of improvement, functional status (activities of daily living), spinal mobility, use of drugs and medical services (2 points each).
N	Each blinded measurement mentioned under point M earns 2 points.
O	Outcome of measures assessed during or just after treatment (3 points). Outcome of measures assessed 6 months or longer (2 points).
P	When loss to follow-up is less than 10%: analysis on all randomized patients for main outcome measures and on the most important points of measurement minus missing values, regardless of noncompliance and co-interventions (5 points). When loss to follow-up is greater than 10%: intention-to-treat as well as an alternative analysis that accounts for missing values (5 points).
Q	For main outcome measures and at main times of measurement: in the case of (semi-) continuous variable, presentation of the mean or median with standard error or centiles (5 points).

Table 2

Number of Studies, by Clinical Condition, Study Design, and Type of Therapy (M=manipulation, m=mobilization)

	Study Design									
	RCT		Cohort		Case Series		Case Report		Total	
Condition	M	m	M	m	M	m	M	m	M	m
Neck Pain										
Acute	0	3	0	0	0	0	3	0	3	3
Subacute/Chronic	5	1	1	1	4	1	21	2	31	5
Total	5	4	1	1	4	1	24	2	34	8
Headache										
Muscle Tension	3 (1)	1	0	0 (1)	7 (1)	0	9 (9)	1 (2)	19 (11)	2 (3)
Migraine	1	0	0	0	2 (2)	0	1	0	4 (2)	0
Total	4	1	0	0	9	0	10	1	23	2
Shoulder/Arm Pain										
Acute/Sub/Chronic	0 (3)	0	0	0 (1)	0 (1)	0	2 (6)	1 (1)	2 (10)	1 (2)
Thoracic Outlet	0 (1)	0	0	0 (1)	0 (1)	3	3 (6)	0	3 (8)	3 (1)
Carpal Tunnel	0	0	0	0	1	0	2 (1)	0	3 (1)	0
Total	0	0	0	0	1	3	7	1	8	4
TMJ Disorders	0	0	0	0	0	0	2 (4)	0 (2)	2 (4)	0 (2)
Other Entities										
BP and HR[a]	1	0	3	0	0	0	0	0	4	0
Cervical Motion	0	0	3	0	2	0	0	0	5	0
Cervical Curvature	0	0	2	0	2	0	0	0	4	0
Miscellaneous	1	0	3	0	5	0	7 (6)	0	16 (6)	0
Total	2	0	11	0	9	0	7	0	29	0
Grand Total	11	5	12	1	23	4	48	4	94	14

Studies employing both manipulation and mobilization are classified under manipulation. Studies having subjects with multiple conditions are numerated in the section corresponding to most subjects' conditions (or, for case reports, the first appropriate condition in the table), then included parenthetically in following sections to avoid multiple counting.

[a]Blood pressure and heart rate.

EFFICACY

The review includes data from 108 studies or reports: 16 RCTs, 13 cohort studies, 27 case series, and 52 case reports. Table 2 presents the number of studies reviewed, classified by clinical condition, research design, and type of therapy.

Table 3 summarizes the RCTs. Table 4 shows the RCTs for neck pain and headache, arranged by descending quality score. The RCTs range in quality from a low of 33 to a high of 77, of a possible 100 points. Most studies scored under 50, which makes these studies similar in quality to the studies of lumbar spine manipulation for low-back pain. For comparison, a recent study of high quality that examined the effect of facet joint injection for back pain (Carette, 1991) scored a 78 using the same criteria.

First priority in the literature search was given to research that used a randomized, controlled trial design (e.g., efficacy). Second priority was given to nonexperimental studies, including cohort, case-control, and cross-sectional studies. Case series and case reports were given lowest priority and were included only for completeness and to document the use of cervical manipulation for conditions for which there was little or no other evidence available. Appropriateness is based on the effectiveness of

Table 3

Randomized Controlled Trials (RCTS) of Cervical Spine Manipulation/Mobilization

Author (Year)	Pain Duration	Case Description	Interventions (n)	Protocol	Results
Neck Pain (Acute)					
Nordemar and Thorner (1981)	< 3 days	Nonradiating cervical pain without neurological symptoms	1)Cervical collar only (10) 2) Collar plus TNS (10) 3) Collar plus traction and mobilization (10)	Groups 2 and 3 received 1 week of 3 treatments by PT	Group 3 had greater increase in mean cervical mobility (132 vs. 65 and 115) and decrease in mean pain (VAS) (79 vs. 55 and 66) after 1 week (P>0.05); no differences between groups at 6 weeks and 3 months.
Mealy et al. (1986)	Not stated	Acute whiplash injury without fracture	1) Maitland mobilization plus exercises (31) 2) Cervical collar plus rest (30)	Group 1 received daily treatment for at least 2 weeks by PT	Mean pain (VAS) less in Group 1 at 4 weeks (2.85 vs. 5.08) and 8 weeks (1.69 vs. 3.94) (P<0.05).and P<0.0125 at 4 and 8 weeks, respectively); greater increase in cervical ROM in Group 1 at 8 weeks (P<0.05).
McKinney (1989). McKinney et al. (1989)	<3 days	Acute flexion-extension sprain without fracture, dislocation, or symptomatic degenerative disease	1) Rest plus analgesics (33) 2) PT modalities plus Maitland mobilization and McKenzie exercises (71) 3) Collar plus advise on mobilization, posture, and exercises (66)	Group 2 received treatments 3 times weekly for 6 weeks by PT	Groups 2 and 3 had greater increases in mean lateral flexion and decreases in pain (VAS) compared to Group 1 after 1 and 2 months (P<0.01); no difference between Groups 2 and 3. A greater proportion of Group 3 subjects were without persistent symptoms at 2 years (77%) compared to Groups 1 (54%) and 2 (56%) (P=0.02).
Neck Pain (Subacute and Chronic)					
Sloop et al. (1982)	> 1 month; mean=6 years (1 month 30 years)	Cervical spondylosis or nonspecific neck pain without progressive neurologic signs	1) Diazepam plus rotational manipulation (21) 2) Diazepam only (18)	Group 1 received 1 treatment given by MD	57% of Group 1 and 28% of Group 2 felt treatment was "helpful" after 3 weeks (P=0.13); trend toward greater pain reduction (VAS) for Group 1 at 3 weeks (5 mm vs. 18 mm improvement) (P=0.20).

Table 3—continued

Neck Pain (Subacute and chronic)					
Author (Year)	Pain Duration	Case Description	Interventions (n)	Protocol	Results
Howe et al. (1983)	Recurrent acute and subacute	Neck, arm, or hand pain from cervical spine lesion with reduced ROM	1) Azapropazone plus rotational manipulation (26) 2) Azapropazone only (26)	Group 1 received 1-3 treatments given by an MD over 1 week	Among neck-pain subjects, 68% of Group 1 and 6% of Group 2 reported subjective pain improvement immediately (P<0.001); no significant differences after 1 and 3 weeks. Immediate increase in cervical rotation in Group 1 maintained at 1 and 3 weeks.
Vernon et al. (1990)	2 weeks-8 years	Chronic mechanical neck pain	1) Rotation manipulation (5) 2) Mobilization (oscillation) (4)	Both groups received 1 treatment given by DC	40-55% rise in pressure pain thresholds around joint fixation immediately in Group 1; no changes in Group 2 (P<0.0001).
Cassidy et al. (1992)	< 1 week (16%) 1 week-6 months (34%) > 6 months (50%)	Unilateral neck pain with referral into trapezius without neurological deficit	1) Rotational manipulation (52) 2) Mobilization (muscle energy (48)	Both groups received 1 treatment given by DC	85% of Group 1 and 69% of Group 2 reported pain improvement (NRS-101) immediately; mean decrease in pain intensity greater in Group 1 (P=0.05; P=0.16 after adjusting for pretreatment differences). ROM increases all greater in Group 1, but none was significant (P>0.05).
Koes et al. (1992, 1993)	> 6 weeks	Nonspecific neck complaint with limited ROM	1) Manipulation and/or mobilization by manual therapists (13) 2) Exercises, massage, and/or modalities by physiotherapists (20) 3) Detuned shortwave diathermy (14) 4) Continued treatment by GP (17)	All groups received treatments for a maximum of 3 months	Greater mean improvement in physical functioning (cervical ROM) in Group 1 compared to Group 2 at 12 weeks (4.8 vs. 3.4), and pain improvement (VAS) at 12 months (4.5 vs. 4.1). No other neck-pain-specific results are provided.

Table 3—continued

Author (Year)	Pain Duration	Case Description	Interventions (n)	Protocol	Results
Neck Pain (Subacute and chronic)					
Brodin (1985)	< 6 months (36%) 6 months-5 years (40%) > 5 years (24%)	Cervical pain with restricted cervical mobility	1) Salicylate only (23) 2) Salicylate plus massage, electrical stimulation, traction, and information ("cervical school") (17) 3) Salicylate and "cervical school," plus passive mobilization (23)	Groups 2 and 3 received 3 treatments weekly for 3 weeks by physiotherapist	Greater proportion of Group 3 subjects had a 30 degree or greater cervical mobility increase at 3 weeks (65% vs. 30% and 35%) ($P<0.001$); less difference 1 week later ($P<0.01$). Group 3 subjects tended to have no or only slight patient-assessed pain 1 week after final treatment (83% vs. 61% and 59%) ($P<0.05$).
Headache (Non-Migraine)					
Hoyt et al. (1979)	Not stated	Muscle contraction headache with history of recurring dull, nonthrobbing bi-lateral headaches without trauma	1) Osteopathic manipulation (10) 2) Palpation only (6) 3) Rest in supine position (6)	Each group received 1 treatment	Mean headache pain decreased within 5 minutes in Group 1 ($P<0.003$); no pre-post changes in Groups 2 and 3.
Jensen et al. (1990)	1 year	Post-traumatic headache	1) Mobilization, manipulation, and muscle energy (10) 2) Cold packs (9)	Each group received 2 treatments 1 week apart	Mean pain index (VAS) decreased to 43% of pretreatment level in Group 1 while there was no change in Group 2, 2 weeks after last treatment (3 weeks from first treatment) ($P<0.05$); pain index increased to 84% of pretreatment level in Group 1, 5 weeks later ($P>0.05$). Frequency of analgesic use and associated symptoms (dizziness, visual disturbances, ear symptoms) decreased nonsignificantly in Group 1 at 8 weeks.

Table 3—continued

Headache (Non-Migraine) (continued)

Author (Year)	Pain Duration	Case Description	Interventions (n)	Protocol	Results
Boline et al. (1994)	> 3 months with at least 1 episode per week	Primarily tension-type headache	1) Spinal manipulation plus moist heat and light massage and OTCs as needed (70) 2) Amitriptyline daily for 6 weeks and OTCs as needed (56)	Group 1 received treatments twice weekly for 6 weeks given by DC: Group 2 was seen at baseline and 6 weeks later	No differences between groups with respect to headache pain intensity, frequency, and OTC use (Blanchard headache diary), or functional status (SF-36), 4 weeks posttreatment, Group 1 had greater than 30% improvements on mean headache intensity, frequency, and OTC use, and a 16% improvement in functional status, while Group 2's changes were under 6%. Differences at 4 weeks include mean headache intensity (3.5 vs. 4.8), frequency (7.2 vs. 10.8), and OTC use (1.2 tablets/day vs. 1.8) (P<0.001), and functional status (78.8 vs. 73.9) (P=0.008).
Carlsson et al. (1990)	Median=7 years (6 months-33 yeas)	Chronic tension headache as part of a fibromyalgic syndrome: all female	1) PT including massage, cryotherapy, TENS, and passive stretching by physiotherapists, plus instruction and exercises (29) 2) Acupuncture (23)	Group 1 received 1-2 sessions per week over 2-3 months; Group 2 received 4-5 treatments over 2-4 weeks	Significant reduction in mean headache intensity (1-5 scale) in Group 1 (3.72 to 2.52, P<0.001) and Group 2 (3.78 to 3.24, P<0.05 for differences between groups. Greater reduction in analgesic intake and muscle tenderness in Group 1 compared to Group 2 (P<0.05). No cervical mobility changes in either group.

Table 3—continued

Headache (Non-Migraine) (continued)

Author (Year)	Pain Duration	Case Description	Interventions (n)	Protocol	Results
Headache (Migraine)					
Parker et al. (1978, 1980)	Mean=19 years	Common (61%) or classical (39%) migraine	1) Manipulation by chiropractor (30) 2) Manipulation by MD or physical therapist (27) 3) Mobilization (oscillation) by MD or physical therapist (28)	Each group received a maximum of 2 months of twice weekly treatments	40% reduction in frequency of attacks and 43% reduction in pain intensity (VAS) in Group 1 from pretreatment to 2 month period posttreatment, compared to 34% and 15% in Group 3 ($P>0.01$). Mean pain intensity less in Group 1 (2.8) compared to Groups 2 (4.4) and 3 (4.5) combined during 2 month posttreatment period ($P<0.01$). No differences with respect to mean frequency of attacks, mean duration of attacks, or mean disability.

Table 4
Quality Scores of Controlled Trials of Manipulation and/or Mobilization of the Cervical Spine*

Neck Pain	Methods Criteria																	
Study (Year)	A 2	B 5	C 4	D 3	E 4	F 12	G 10	H 5	I 5	J 5	K 5	L 5	M 10	N 10	O 5	P 5	Q 5	Total 100
Koes et al. (1992)	1	4	2	3	2	6	3	5	4	5	4	3	8	8	5	5	5	73
Cassidy et al. (1992)	1	5	2	3	4	0	10	0	0	0	5	0	4	4	3	5	5	51
Sloop et al. (1982)	1	1	2	0	4	0	5	0	0	5	5	5	4	4	3	5	5	49
Nordemar et al. (1981)	1	3	1	3	4	0	5	5	5	0	0	0	4	0	3	5	5	44
Howe et al. (1983)	1	3	2	3	4	0	5	5	0	0	0	0	4	2	3	5	5	42
Brodin (1985)	1	1	4	3	4	0	10	5	0	0	0	0	4	0	3	0	5	40
McKinney et al. (1989)	1	2	1	3	0	0	5	5	0	5	0	0	4	4	3	0	5	38
Vernon et al. (1990)	0	1	2	0	4	0	5	0	0	0	5	3	2	2	3	5	5	37
Mealy et al. (1986)	1	2	4	3	2	0	0	5	0	0	0	0	4	4	3	0	5	33
Headache																		
Boline et al. (1994)	2	5	4	3	3	6	10	5	5	0	5	0	8	8	3	5	5	77
Parker et al. (1978)	2	5	2	3	4	0	5	0	0	0	5	2	6	6	5	5	5	55
Jensen et al. (1990)	2	5	2	3	2	0	5	5	5	0	0	3	6	6	3	0	5	52
Hoyt et al. (1979)	2	1	2	0	4	0	5	0	0	5	5	3	2	2	3	5	0	39
Carlsson et al. (1990)	1	3	2	3	2	0	5	0	0	0	0	0	6	6	3	0	5	36

*Refer to Table 1 for definitions of the letters, A through Q.

the procedure as performed by the average practitioner in the community. Because hardly any published comparative studies were found of the use of cervical spine manipulation or mobilization that have used a community-based practitioner sample, for the purposes of informing this panel, we had to rely on studies of efficacy. The two are related, however, for without efficacy, there can be no effectiveness.

In interpreting this report, several points should be kept in mind. First, the quality of the studies is extremely variable. Ideally, all studies would use a randomized design in which the manipulation is allocated to the study population so that everyone has an equal probability of receiving the manipulation or the control procedure. This process, by helping to ensure comparability between treatment groups, prevents confounding by prognostic factors for the outcome (e.g., pain reduction), provided that the study population is large enough. Because of potential selection bias and confounding, it is impossible to make efficacy determinations using nonrandomized studies and studies without a comparison group (case series and case reports). For example, subjects in case series or case reports may have resolved equally well on their own or may have had a quicker recovery or a better outcome with another treatment. The randomized controlled trials are listed in Table 3. The quality scoring of the controlled trials is shown in Table 4. The significance of a difference between studies of a few points in quality scores is not known, but large differences in quality scores between studies reflect real differences in study design, execution, and reporting. It is assumed that better scoring studies are less prone to bias and are therefore more likely to report valid results.

Second, to minimize measurement error and misclassification, the outcome should be valid, reliable, and assessed by an examiner who is blind to exposure status. The outcomes, especially in the case series and case reports, were subjectively (and often unclearly) defined, were of unknown reliability and validity, and were often assessed by an unblinded investigator. In addition, the clinical significance of outcome measures such as cervical range of motion is not well established, and similar variables (e.g., degrees of straight-leg raising) have been shown to correlate poorly with functional status in patients with low-back pain (Deyo, 1988). When pain is reported, it is frequently measured using a visual analogue scale (VAS) that asks the patient to place a mark on a 100-millimeter line anchored by "no pain" and "worst pain ever."

Third, the study populations were often comprised of subjects with a variety of symptom complexes (e.g., neck pain with and without arm pain, migraine and tension headache) and with inherently different prognoses (e.g., acute and chronic pain, traumatic and nontraumatic neck pain). Ideally, study populations would be comprised of subjects with symptoms of similar etiologies and similar prognoses. Alternatively, if sample sizes are large enough, investigators could stratify on etiologic or prognostic factors and perform analyses within each stratum. However, sample sizes were generally too small to employ this strategy. Fourth, because spinal manipulation is a term used for many techniques, the manual procedure should be described explicitly. It was often difficult (or impossible) to discern the type of manipulation, the location (i.e., which joints of the cervical spine), and the duration (number of treatments and total time) of care. Furthermore, many studies employed multiple treatments within the manipulation (or mobilization) groups, making it difficult to assess the independent effect of manipulation (or mobilization).

Finally, it would have been informative to have been able to combine data from different studies. Unfortunately, this was not possible due to investigators using heterogeneous outcome measures, including subjects with acute and chronic pain (and not reporting results separately for each), and assessing outcomes at different post-treatment times.

For the purposes of this review, acute pain is defined as pain of less than three weeks' duration; subacute pain is that of three to 13 weeks' duration; and chronic pain is pain lasting longer than 13 weeks. Studies employing both manipulation and mobilization are classified under manipulation.

NECK PAIN

Five RCTs, one cohort study, four case series, and 24 case reports were identified that attempted to assess the effectiveness of cervical spine manipulation for the treatment of neck pain. An additional four RCTs, one cohort study, and one case series dealt with, at least in part, the effectiveness of mobilization for neck pain. The manipulation RCTs focused primarily on subacute and chronic pain, whereas three of the mobilization RCTs addressed acute pain. The quality scores of these studies ranged from 33 to 73.

Acute Neck Pain

Randomized controlled trials (manipulation). Howe et al. (1983), Vernon et al. (1990), and Cassidy et al. (1992b) conducted randomized studies assessing the efficacy of cervical spine manipulation for neck pain. The majority of subjects in each trial were suffering from recurrent, subacute, or chronic pain, but the trials included acute pain subjects. The investigators did not stratify their results by duration of pain.

Randomized controlled trials (mobilization). Nordemar and Thorner (1981) received the highest quality score (44) among studies designed to test the effect of mobilization against other therapies for acute neck pain. Thirty patients with non-radiating cervical pain of less than three days' duration were randomized into three groups: (1) neck collar only (n=10); (2) collar plus transcutaneous electrical nerve stimulation (TENS) (n=10); and (3) collar plus manual therapy consisting of soft tissue, traction, mobilization, and static muscle work against resistance delivered by a physiotherapist (n=10). After one week of three treatments, the manual therapy group had higher mean improvements in cervical mobility and pain reduction (as measured by a visual-analogue scale), which were not statistically different from the other groups (P>0.05). No differences between groups were detected at six weeks and three months. The small sample size and high degree of variability among the outcome measures between subjects within each group may have masked any differences between groups.

McKinney (1989a) received a relatively low quality score of 38. One-hundred-seventy subjects were assessed within 72 hours from suffering acute flexion-extension neck sprains. Subjects were randomized into one of three groups: (1) rest and analgesics (n=33); (2) six weeks of treatments including physical therapy modalities plus Maitland movements delivered by a physiotherapist and McKenzie exercises (n=71); or (3) neck collar plus advice on mobilization, posture and exercises (n=66). Groups 2 and 3 had significant increases in mean goniometer-assessed lateral flexion (P<0.01) and decreases in VAS-assessed pain severity after one and two months, which were significantly different from Group 1, but not different from each other. A greater proportion of Group 3 subjects were without persistent symptoms at two years (77 percent) compared to Groups 1 (54 percent) and 2 (56 percent) (P=0.02).

Among all trials assessing the effect of mobilization or manipulation for neck pain, Mealy et al. (1986) received the lowest quality score (33). Mealy's team studied 61 patients who had suffered acute whiplash injuries. Subjects were randomized into groups that received Maitland mobilization delivered by a physiotherapist and daily exercises (n=31) or cervical collar (n=30). Mean VAS-based pain intensity was significantly less in the mobilization group at four weeks (P<0.05) and eight weeks (P<0.0125). Although both groups showed goniometer-assessed range-of-motion increases at four weeks, only the mobilization group's increase was statistically significant, and at eight weeks, the mobilization group's range of motion increase was significantly greater than the collar group's increase (P<0.05).

In summary, there are no RCTs or case series presenting data about the efficacy of cervical spine manipulation specifically for patients with acute neck pain. The limited literature available on mobilization for acute neck pain indicates that it may be beneficial for some patients, at least compared to rest and cervical collar, although instruction on mobilization and exercises may be equally beneficial.

Subacute and Chronic Neck Pain

Randomized controlled trials (manipulation). Koes et al. (1992a,b,c, 1993) received the highest quality score by our raters (73) among studies with subjects having subacute or chronic neck pain. The quality score may be somewhat misleading, however, since only a small subset of subjects in the studies had neck pain. Koes et al. (1992c) studied 64 patients with nonspecific neck complaints as part of a larger study assessing the effectiveness of manual therapy for chronic (duration longer than six weeks) nonspecific back and neck complaints. Subjects were randomized into one of four treatment groups: (1) manual therapy including manipulation and mobilization delivered by manual and physical therapists (n=13); (2) physical therapy only (n=20), (3) placebo (detuned shortwave diathermy) (n=14); and (4) usual general practitioner care (n=17). Each assigned treatment was given for a maximum of three months. Unfortunately, the authors combined back and neck complaints for most of their analyses. For back and neck complaints together, improvements in severity of the main complaint and in physical functioning were larger with manipulative therapy and mobilization than with physiotherapy (consisting of exercise, massage, and/or other modalities). The following results are the ones available for neck complaints only. At 12 weeks, the mean improvement in the main complaint, based on a 10-point VAS, was 4.5 for the manual therapy group (n=12) and 4.1 for the physical therapy group (n=17). At 12 weeks, the mean improvement in physical functioning, based on cervical range of motion, was 4.8 for the manual therapy group (n=12) and 3.4 for the physical therapy group (n=17). Inferential statistics were not computed, and necessary data for their computation were not provided.

Cassidy et al. (1992a) received the second highest quality score (51) in this group. They studied 100 subjects suffering from unilateral neck pain with referral into the trapezius. Sixteen subjects had been in pain for less than one week; 34, for one week to six months; and 50, for longer than six months. Subjects were randomized to one of two groups: (1) one rotational manipulation delivered by a chiropractor or (2) one session of mobilization (muscle energy technique). Immediately after the intervention, 85 percent of the manipulated group reported pain improvement while 69 percent of the mobilized group reported improvement. The mean decrease in pain intensity, based on the 101-point numerical rating scale (NRS-101), decreased 17.3 points in the manipulated group versus 10.5 points in the mobilization group (P=0.05; P=0.16 after adjusting for pretreatment differences). Range of motion increases were all greater in the manipulated group, but none was statistically significant (P>0.05).

Sloop et al. (1982), which received a quality score of 49, studied 39 patients with cervical spondylosis or nonspecific neck pain (37 also had arm pain) who had been suffering for at least one month (6 years was the average). Twenty-one patients were randomized to receive diazepam and one rotational manipulation given by an M.D. while 18 received diazepam only. After three weeks, 12/21 (57 percent) of the manipulated group and 5/18 (28 percent) of the diazepam-only group felt the treatment was helpful (P=0.13). At 12 weeks, the figures were 7/9 (78 percent) and 2/6 (33 percent), respectively (P=0.17). There were no statistically significant differences on a visual-analogue scale (VAS), but there was a greater trend toward improvement in the manipulated group (P=0.20). This study may not have had enough power to detect a difference between the treatment groups because only 39 subjects were studied.

Howe et al. (1983) received a quality score of 42. They studied 52 patients who had neck, arm, or hand pain thought to be caused by a lesion of the cervical spine. Forty-one (79 percent) had suffered for more than four weeks. Twenty-six were randomly assigned to receive azapropazone plus one to three rotational manipulations delivered by an M.D., while 26 were assigned to receive azapropazone only. Of the patients with neck pain, 13/19 (68 percent) of the manipulated group and 1/17 (6 percent) of the control group improved immediately based on patients' subjective report of pain improvement (P<0.001). Of the patients with pain or paresthesia of the shoulder (n=39), 10/22 (45 percent) of the manipulated group and 1/17 (6 percent) of the control group showed immediate improvement (P<0.02). Among subjects with pain or paresthesia of the arm or hand, 6/12 (50 percent) of the manipulated group and 1/9 (11 percent) of the control group showed immediate improvement, while at one week, 9/12 (75 percent) and 4/7 (57 percent) showed improvement, respectively. Although these differences between groups are not statistically significant (P>0.05), they do show a trend toward a positive effect for manipulation. No significant differences in subjective pain status between groups were detected after one and three weeks; however, cervical rotation immediately increased in the manipulated group, and this was maintained at each assessment (assessed by a goniometer read by an examiner blind to exposure status).

Vernon et al. (1990) received the second lowest quality score (37) among the neck pain trials. Nine subjects with chronic mechanical neck pain who had been suffering from two weeks to eight years were studied. Five subjects were randomly assigned to receive one rotational manipulation delivered by a chiropractor, while four subjects were randomized to a mobilization (oscillation technique) group. Pressure pain threshold (PPT) readings were taken at four points surrounding the joint fixation by an examiner blind to exposure status before and after manipulation or mobilization. Immediately after the intervention, there was a 40 to 55 percent rise in PPT for all four points around the fixation for the manipulated group, whereas no changes were shown for the mobilization group ($P<0.0001$).

Randomized controlled trials (mobilization). Brodin (1985), with a quality score of 40, conducted a study with 63 cervical pain subjects who had been suffering from fewer than six months (36.5 percent) to more than five years (24 percent). Subjects were randomized into one of three groups: (1) salicylate only (n=23), (2) salicylate plus massage, electrical muscle stimulation, traction, and general back information (n=17), or (3) salicylate, information, plus manual mobilization of specific cervical spine segments (n=23). Subjects in Groups 2 and 3 were treated three times weekly for three weeks by a physiotherapist. At three weeks from baseline, a greater proportion of Group 3 subjects (65 percent) had a 30 degree or greater increase in cervical mobility, compared to Groups 1 (30 percent) and 2 (35 percent) ($P<0.001$). This difference became statistically nonsignificant a week later ($P<0.1$). A greater proportion of Group 3 subjects (83 percent) had no pain or only slight patient-assessed pain one week after the final treatment, compared to Groups 1 (61 percent) and 2 (59 percent) ($P<0.05$).

Other studies. Arkuszewski (1986) performed a cohort study of 100 subjects with lumbago or sciatica (60 percent also had neck pain) in which 50 received manual treatment administered by a manual therapist consisting of traction, mobilization and/or manipulation, and muscle energy to all parts of the spine, and 50 received standard drug treatment and physical therapy. Treatments were twice weekly for an unspecified period. The author reported that neurological symptoms, posture, and intensity of pain (all measured on 0–3 scales) showed greater improvement in patients in the manual therapy group at discharge and six months later. All 100 patients contributed data to the discharge outcome measurement, whereas 88 patients had outcomes measured at six months.

Livingston (1969) reported on a case series of 64 consecutive patients of which eight had neck pain. One year after receiving two to 15 treatments of cervical manipulation (M.D.-administered, Cyriax-style), two reported "excellent" results (no symptoms), one reported a "good" result (more than 90 percent better), four were improved (50 to 90 percent better), and one reported no change in symptoms.

Beal et al. (1989) reported a case series of four patients with motion impairment and chronic cervical pain of at least six weeks' duration following a cervical spine injury. After three months of weekly osteopathic treatments (soft tissue and manipulation, if indicated), all four subjects had improved EMG readings, palpatory findings, and subjective pain improvement.

Mennell (1990) reported a case series of 100 patients with neck (n=50), arm (n=13), shoulder (n=7), or head pain or headaches (n=23), of duration ranging from zero days to more than one year (n=61). Eighty-three were manipulated by an M.D. (32 were manipulated under anesthesia). Of the 37 neck-pain patients who were manipulated, after an average follow-up of two years, 15 were "cured" (complete freedom from symptoms), 13 reported "marked improvement," seven reported "moderate improvement," and two had no change in symptoms. All seven patients with shoulder pain had moderate or marked improvement, while 11/12 (92 percent) of the arm-pain patients were either improved or "cured" (one patient was unchanged).

Cassidy et al. (1992b) reported on a series of 50 consecutive patients with unilateral neck pain without neurological deficit. Twenty percent had been suffering for less than one week, 30 percent from one week to six months, and 50 percent had been in pain for more than six months. Five minutes after one chiropractor-administered cervical rotational manipulation, cervical range of motion increased in all planes and post-treatment pain-intensity scores (based on the 101-point numerical rating scale) decreased from a pretreatment mean of 43.7 to a post-treatment mean of 31.1. Thirty-seven patients (74 percent) reported improvement in their pain, whereas five patients (10 percent) reported an increase in their pain within five minutes after the treatment.

Graff-Radford et al. (1987) reported on a series of 25 patients referred to a pain management center with head and neck pain of durations ranging from one to 50 years (mean=11.25 years). All subjects had deep, dull aches with active myofascial trigger points and no symptoms suggesting vascular, neurogenic, organic, or psychologic etiology. Patients received an outline and rationale for a multidisciplinary approach to care: exercises; education on posture, stress management and relaxation; medication reduction, and myofascial pain and physical therapy (cervical mobilization, traction, heat, ultrasound, and/or massage) twice weekly for six weeks; plus spray and stretch once weekly for six weeks. Significant reductions were reported in medication intake and self-rated pain using a visual-analogue scale after six weeks ($P<0.001$), which were maintained at three-, six-, and twelve-month follow-ups.

Rundcrantz et al. (1991) performed a cohort study among 44 dentists with one to two years of occupational headache and neck and shoulder pain. Twenty-two subjects received ergonomic instruction only and 22 received ergonomic instruction and home exercises plus one to eight physical therapy sessions consisting of stretching, mobilization, and traction delivered by a physiotherapist. After five weeks from baseline, the physical therapy group demonstrated a significant decrease in mean VAS-assessed neck pain ($P<0.05$) and improvement in VAS-assessed overall well-being ($P<0.05$), while no pre-post changes were detected in the ergonomic instruction group.

In summary, evidence from the literature supports the conclusion that cervical spine manipulation and/or mobilization may provide at least short-term pain relief and range of motion enhancement for persons with subacute or chronic neck pain. The published results are insufficient to make efficacy determinations separately for patients with subacute pain and patients with chronic neck pain.

HEADACHE

Five RCTs, 10 case series, and 19 case reports were identified that assessed the effectiveness of cervical spine manipulation for headache. One additional RCT addressed, in part, the effectiveness of mobilization techniques for headache. One of the RCTs (Parker et al., 1978, 1980), two of the case series (Wight, 1978; Stodolny and Chmielewski, 1989), and one of the case reports (Fitzgerald, 1991) assessed the effectiveness of manipulation for migraine sufferers. The other case series may have included common or classical migraine sufferers among their cases. The quality scores of the RCTs ranged from 36 to 77.

Muscle Tension Headache

Randomized controlled trials (manipulation). Boline et al. (1994) received the highest quality score (77) among the RCTs evaluated in this review. The results of this study have been presented at several scientific meetings but are currently unpublished. The following information is taken from the manuscript submitted to a peer-reviewed journal. Subjects with tension-type headaches of at least three months' duration and with not less than one episode per week were randomized into one of two groups: (1) spinal manipulation performed by a chiropractor, plus moist heat and light massage (n=70), or (2) amitriptyline daily for six weeks (n=56). Each subject in the manipulation group received treatments twice weekly for six weeks, while amitriptyline subjects were seen only at baseline and six weeks later. Both groups were allowed to take over-the-counter medications (OTCs) as needed. Two previously validated instruments were used to assess outcomes: the Blanchard headache diary was used to assess pain intensity, headache frequency, and over-the-counter drug use; the SF-36 was used to assess functional status. After the six-week treatment period, no differences were detected between groups with respect to headache pain intensity, frequency, OTC use, or functional status. Four weeks later, Group 1 subjects had improvements from baseline on headache intensity (32 percent reduction), frequency (37 percent reduction), over-the-counter drug use (37 percent reduction), and functional status (16 percent improvement), whereas all improvements in Group 2 were less than six percent. In addition, differences were detected between groups with respect to mean headache intensity (3.5 vs. 4.8), frequency (7.2 vs. 10.8), over-the-counter use (1.2 tablets/day vs. 1.8) ($P<0.001$), and functional status (78.8 vs. 73.9) ($P=0.008$).

Jensen et al. (1990) received a quality score of 52 by the reviewers in this current study. Twenty-three patients suffering from post-traumatic headache one year following the trauma were assigned by randomization to receive manual therapy (mobilization, cervical and/or upper thoracic manipulation, and muscle energy) or cold packs. Patients in each group were treated twice and could concurrently take analgesics. Nineteen subjects completed the study. Two weeks after the final treatment, the mean pain index (VAS) was 43 percent of the pretreatment level in the manual therapy group, whereas virtually no change occurred in the cold pack group (P<0.05 for difference between groups). Five weeks later, the mean pain index in the manual therapy group was 84 percent of the pretreatment level, which is not statistically different from pretreatment level or from the cold pack group (P>0.05).

The Hoyt et al. (1979) study, which received the lowest quality score (39) by the current reviewers in this group, randomized 22 patients with muscle contraction headache and a history of dull, nonthrobbing bilateral headaches recurring over months or years with posterior cervical discomfort to one of three groups: (1) osteopathic manipulation, including deep pressure, stretching, and high-velocity manipulation (n=10); (2) palpatory examination only (n=6), or (3) rest in a supine position (n=6). All treatments lasted ten minutes. The authors reported a statistically significant reduction in rated headache pain within five minutes after treatment in the manipulation group (P<0.0003) and no changes in the other groups. The authors also reported no pre-post changes in EMG readings or dominant hand temperatures, and no differences between groups.

Howe et al. (1983) included 27 subjects with headache in their RCT comparing manipulation and azapropazone (n=14) with azapropazone only (n=13) and received a score of 62 from the raters. No statistically significant differences were found in proportion of subjects showing improvement between groups at any of the three assessments (immediately after treatment and one and three weeks later). However, with the small sample size for this subgroup analysis, even a relatively large difference would not demonstrate statistical significance.

Randomized controlled trials (mobilization). Carlsson et al. (1990) received the lowest quality score (36) among the headache trials. These researchers conducted a trial with female tension headache sufferers who had been in pain for six months to 33 years (median=7 years). Subjects were randomized into groups receiving either (1) physiotherapy including instruction, massage, cryotherapy, Transcutaneous Electrical Nerve Stimulation (TENS), passive stretching, relaxation, and exercises (n=29) or (2) acupuncture (n=23). The physiotherapy group received one to two sessions per week over two to three months, while the acupuncture group received four to five treatments over a two to four week period, with an option of four to five additional treatments. Significant reductions were reported in mean headache intensity (measured on a 1–5 scale) in Group 1 (3.72 to 2.52, P<0.001) and Group 2 (3.78 to 3.24, P<0.05); P<0.05 for the difference between groups. In addition, there was a greater reduction in analgesic intake and muscle tenderness in Group 1 compared to Group 2 (P<0.05). Cervical spine mobility remained unchanged in both groups from pretreatment to post-treatment.

Other studies. Livingston (1969) reported a case series of 64 patients who were treated with Cyriax-style traction manipulation of the cervical spine. Of the eight cervical syndrome cases that are documented in some detail, seven reported positive results and one reported no change after one year of from two to 15 treatments. A whiplash case was "improved" (50 to 90 percent better) after eight treatments and a migraine patient reported "good" results (more than 90 percent better) with decreased severity and frequency of attacks after 13 treatments.

Lewit (1977) described a case series of 64 subjects with cervical headache (n=24), migrainous attacks (n=21), or pain on flexion or extension (n=19). Six or more months after treatment with manipulation (delivered by a manual therapist), needling or infiltration with anesthetics, or massage (nine patients were treated with manipulation only), 33 had "excellent" results, 22 had "good" results, and there were nine "failures" (five of these were migraine sufferers).

Schultz (1977) reported that of the five patients who participated in a case series of headache subjects and received osteopathic manipulation, all were made worse (assessed by patient self-report).

Vernon (1982b) conducted a study of 33 subjects (15 retrospectively, 18 prospectively) with benign cervicogenic cephalgia or migraine, ranging in duration from less than one to 30 years, who were treated with chiropractic adjustments. Statistically significant ($P<0.01$) reductions in headache frequency, duration, and pain severity were found after an average of 12 visits in the retrospective group and nine visits in the prospective group. In addition, no side effects were reported, and associated symptoms such as nausea, dizziness, tinnitus, and aura were relieved in most patients.

Droz and Krot (1985) reported the results of a series of 332 patients with occipital headaches who were treated with an average of 8.6 chiropractic treatments. Two hundred sixty-four had "good" or "excellent" outcomes (pain-free or almost pain-free); 33 (10 percent) had a 75 percent decrease in symptoms; 17 (5 percent) were the same or only slightly better; and symptoms were aggravated in 17 (5 percent) of the patients.

Jirout (1985) described a case series of 200 patients with C2-C3 rotation restrictions (90 percent had headaches in the occipital region) who underwent one or two treatments of cervical manipulation and/or postisometric relaxation delivered by a manual therapist. All cases had their restrictions removed; 107 (53.5 percent) "felt better"; 35 (17.5 percent) reported no symptoms; and 47 (23.5 percent) were lost to follow-up.

Turk and Ratkolb (1987) reported the results of a case series of 100 patients with chronic cervicogenous headaches who were treated by a manual therapist with specific manipulations of the cervical spine twice weekly for three weeks. After one week, 56 patients' headaches decreased to half of their pretreatment level, and 75 decreased to half after three weeks. Six months later, 25 said they had no headaches, whereas 40 were "improved" but still took analgesics. In 35 patients, improvement had occurred for a month, but headaches recurred again within six months.

Mennell (1990) had 23 patients with headache of duration ranging from one week to 41 years in his case series of cervical subjects. Of the 20 patients who were manipulated, after an average follow-up of two years, five (25 percent) were free of symptoms, six (30 percent) had "marked improvement," seven (35 percent) had "moderate improvement," and two (10 percent) had no change.

A study by Rundcrantz et al. (1991) comparing manual therapy to ergonomic instruction among dentists demonstrated a statistically nonsignificant attenuation of VAS-assessed headache pain among dentists in the manual therapy group, while no prepost difference was reported in the ergonomic instruction group [see p.20, Subacute and Chronic Neck Pain, for more details].

In summary, the literature is sparse but suggests that cervical spine manipulation and/or mobilization may provide short-term relief for some patients with muscle tension (and other nonmigraine) headaches. The evidence for long-term benefit is much less conclusive.

Migraine Headache

Randomized controlled trial (manipulation). The Parker et al. (1978, 1980) studies, which received the third highest quality score (55) of RCTs in this review, conducted a trial in which 85 migraine sufferers (61 percent common, 39 percent classical) were randomized into one of three groups: (1) chiropractic manipulation (n=30), (2) manipulation performed by an M.D. or physical therapist (n=27), or (3) mobilization performed by an M.D. or physical therapist (n=28). After a two-month period of no more than two treatments per week, chiropractors were more likely to assess treatment as useful and appropriate and to regard further treatment as necessary. Chiropractic patients reported a 40 percent reduction in frequency of attacks and a 43 percent reduction in pain intensity (based on a VAS), compared with 34 percent and 15 percent in Group 3 ($P<0.01$). In addition, they reported less mean pain intensity compared to Groups 2 and 3 combined during the two-month post-treatment period ($P<0.01$). No differences were detected with respect to mean frequency of attacks, mean duration of attacks, or mean disability. However, of the 14 patients who reported no migraine attacks, eight were chiropractic patients; five of the six others were mobilization patients. After 20 months, of the 14/73 (19 percent) subjects who reported no attacks during the preceding two months, eight were chiropractic patients, two were M.D. manipulation patients, and four were from the mobilization group. This is a significant difference ($p<0.05$) between the chiropractors and the medical manipulators but not between the chiropractors and the mobilization group.

Other studies. Wight (1978) reported on a series of common (n=34) and classical (n=53) migraine sufferers. Subjects were given from 1 to 74 chiropractic adjustments, usually on a weekly basis. Two years after the final treatments, a questionnaire was administered to each subject. Of the common migraine sufferers, 24 (70.6 percent) "improved" and 10 (29.4 percent) did not improve (two became worse). Of the classical migraine sufferers, 41 (77.4 percent) "improved," and 12 (22.6 percent) did not improve (two became worse). Common migraine sufferers had a 62.6 percent reduction in number of headaches from the year preceding treatment compared to the year following treatment, whereas classical migraine sufferers had a 39.2 percent reduction.

Stodolny and Chmielewski (1989) conducted a case series of 31 patients with cervical migraine (mean duration 8.3 years) who were treated with cervical manipulation and mobilization by a manual therapist. Headache intensity and cervical spine pain intensity were measured on 0–4 scales immediately following treatment and seven days later. Mean headache-intensity scores decreased from 2.35 to 1.71 to 0.94 seven days later, whereas mean cervical-spine pain-intensity scores decreased from 2.03 to 1.74 to 1.06 seven days later. Cervical range of motion increased from a mean of 136 to 154.2 immediately after treatment, then regressed to 147.9 seven days later.

Livingston (1969), Lewit (1977), and Vernon (1982b) included subjects with migraine or migrainous attacks in their studies. Although results were not stratified by type of headache, Lewit reported that five of the nine "failures" in his study were migraine sufferers.

In summary, the literature is too limited to support or refute the use of cervical spine manipulation and/or mobilization for patients suffering from migraine headaches.

SHOULDER/ARM/HAND PAIN

Acute, Subacute, and Chronic Pain

Randomized controlled trials (manipulation). The RCTs of Sloop et al. (1982), Howe et al. (1983), and Cassidy et al. (1992a) (whose rating scores were shown previously as 42 and 51 respectively) included subjects with shoulder and/or arm pain [see p. 20, Subacute and Chronic Neck Pain]; however, since only Howe stratified data on pain location, very limited conclusions can be drawn with respect to the efficacy of cervical spine manipulation for shoulder and/or arm pain.

Among the patients with pain or paresthesia of the shoulder (n=39), 10/22 (45 percent) of the manipulated group and 1/17 (6 percent) of the control group showed immediate improvement ($P<0.02$). Among subjects with pain or paresthesia of the arm or hand, 6/12 (50 percent) of the manipulated group and 1/9 (11 percent) of the control group showed immediate improvement, whereas at one week, 9/12 (75 percent) and 4/7 (57 percent) showed improvement, respectively. Although these differences between groups are not statistically significant ($P>0.05$), they do show a trend toward a positive effect for manipulation.

Other studies. Mennell's (1990) case series included 13 patients with arm pain and seven patients with shoulder pain. All seven patients with shoulder pain had "moderate" or "marked" improvement, whereas 11/12 (92 percent) of the arm-pain patients were either "improved" or "cured" (one patient was unchanged). The Rundcrantz et al. study (1991) of dentists with cervicobrachial pain of 12 to 24 months duration found that shoulder pain was not significantly reduced after five weeks among those who received one to eight treatments of cervical traction, mobilization, stretching, home exercises, and ergonomic instruction.

In summary, the literature is insufficient to support or refute the use of cervical spine manipulation and/or mobilization for patients with pain of the shoulder, arm, and/or hand of any duration.

Thoracic Outlet Syndrome

No RCTs, cohort studies, or case series were found that explicitly address the effectiveness of cervical spine manipulation or mobilization for the treatment of thoracic outlet or related syndromes. Three case series describe the use of mobilization techniques for thoracic outlet conditions, whereas three case reports address the use of manipulation. Subjects with arm pain or paresthesias in the studies assessing the effect of cervical spine manipulation for neck pain and headache may have been suffering from thoracic outlet problems (Howe et al., 1983; Mennell, 1990; Rundcrantz et al., 1991). In addition, many of the neck-pain case reports also involved arm pain or paresthesias (A. M. Robertson, 1968; J. A. Robertson, 1978; Hammond, 1983; Vernon, 1988; Mariano et al., 1991; Siciliano et al., 1992).

Case series (mobilization). Smith (1979) describes a case series of 20 patients with paresthesias, numbness, and pain who received information on posture and exercises and were treated 1 to 14 times by a physical therapist with mobilization, stretching, massage, and cervical traction. Fifteen subjects (75 percent) reported "improvement" (fewer, less severe, or only occasional episodes) following care. After an additional one month to two years, 11 of these improvers reported no recurrence or regression.

Sallstrom and Celegin (1983) described 99 patients with thoracic outlet syndrome who had been suffering for one month to 12 years. Seventeen had previous neck-shoulder trauma, including 12 whiplash cases. The patients were given exercise instruction and posture training plus ultrasound, heat, and soft-tissue mobilization delivered by a physiotherapist. Of the patients with slight or moderate symptoms (e.g., positional paresthesias, intermittent cervicobrachial pain), 53/66 (80 percent) had a "good" or "excellent" outcome, while only 3/33 (12 percent) of the subjects with severe symptoms (e.g., partially incapacitated from pain or paresthesias) had a similar outcome. The mean duration of symptoms in responders was 1.5 years versus 4.3 years in nonresponders. In addition, 15/17 (88 percent) of the trauma patients had "poor" results.

Ingesson et al. (1986) described a series of 125 subjects with chronic thoracic outlet symptoms (duration of symptoms ranging from two months to 22 years) who received one to eight sessions of education, relaxation, and physiotherapist-administered cervical and thoracic mobilization over six to eight weeks. After the treatment period, 63/125 (50 percent) had a "good" or "fair" result (e.g., reduction of pain, numbness, and/or tingling), while 62/125 (50 percent) had a "poor" result. The mean duration of symptoms was significantly shorter in responders (12 months) compared to nonresponders (24 months) ($P<0.01$). Also, responders were somewhat less likely to have had trauma (20/63 or 32 percent) compared to nonresponders (27/62 or 44 percent) ($P>0.01$).

Case reports (manipulation). Grice (1977) documented a case of scalenus anticus syndrome in which the patient had pain over shoulder, upper arm, medial side of forearm, thumb, and forefinger. After an anterior cervical adjustment, the patient had dramatic pain relief. Glick (1989) documented a case of cervicobrachalgia where the patient suffered with upper cervical pain radiating into left arm and lateral thorax and paresthesias of C5, C6, and C7 dermatomes of one week duration following a ski fall. After one chiropractic adjustment to the cervical spine, the patient experienced noticeable relief and increased range of motion. Complete symptom resolution occurred after the third visit. Greenly and Bergmann (1990) reported a case of teres syndrome where the patient experienced left shoulder pain and weakness following a motor vehicle accident. The patient experienced pain-free shoulder abduction and normal strength after specific adjustments to C5-6, shoulder adjustments, heat, stretching, and Codman pendulum exercises.

In summary, there is insufficient evidence to support or refute the use of cervical spine manipulation and/or mobilization for patients with thoracic outlet syndrome. The literature indicates that manipulation and mobilization may be more effective in patients with acute or subacute symptoms.

CARPAL TUNNEL SYNDROME

No RCTs or cohort studies were found that assess the effectiveness of cervical spine manipulation or mobilization for treatment of carpal tunnel syndrome. One case series and two case reports were found in the literature.

Case series (manipulation). Bonebrake et al. (1990,1993) described a case series of 43 carpal tunnel cases (only 25 patients completed the study) who were treated with hard-tissue chiropractic manipulation to the cervical, thoracic, and lumbar spines and extremities; soft-tissue manipulation; dietary modifications; exercises; and in some cases, ultrasound. After an average treatment duration of 45 days (4 to 162 day range) with an average of 27 treatments (3 to 96 range), there were some statistically significant strength and range of motion increases, as well as a 15 percent average decrease in pain and distress rating among the 25 who completed the study. An evaluation of 22 of the 25 subjects six months later found that grip strength, EMG, and range of motion increases were maintained.

Case reports (manipulation). Valente (1991) documented the case of a carpal tunnel patient with pain, tingling, and numbness of hands, pain in wrists, tingling in forearms and elbows, and neck pain. The patient felt better after two months of extremity and spinal manipulative therapy delivered by a chiropractor, splinting, ice, ultrasound, and vitamin B6. The patient had a negative EMG and experienced a "significant" decrease in pain and tingling two months later but continued to have pain, numbness, and tingling during work.

Mariano et al. (1991) described a patient with left lower cervical and upper thoracic pain, radiation into left arm with numbness and paresthesias into left hand. An EMG revealed C6-C7 radiculopathy and moderate carpal tunnel syndrome with mild denervation. Six months after treatment with spinal manipulative therapy and mobilization of the cervical spine delivered by a chiropractor, ultrasound, electrical nerve stimulation, home traction, and wrist splint, the patient experienced only occasional intermittent minimal symptoms of neck and arm pain with paresthesia.

In summary, there is insufficient evidence to support or refute the use of cervical spine manipulation and/or mobilization for patients with carpal tunnel syndrome.

TMJ DISORDERS

There are no RCTs, cohort studies, or case series reporting the effectiveness of cervical spine manipulation or mobilization in the treatment of TMJ disorders. Eight case reports are documented in the literature, six using manipulation and two using mobilization.

Case reports (manipulation). Burns (1979) described two cases of patients with jaw aches who were "improved" after each having one cervical manipulation. Nykoliation and Cassidy (1984) described two cases. One patient experienced pain over both TMJs for years and frequent headaches. After three days of once-daily manipulations to the TMJ and upper cervical facets, the patient experienced a 40 percent "improvement," and after several months of twice-weekly manipulations, the patient was virtually pain-free. The second patient had left jaw pain and neck stiffness for four months. The patient experienced temporary relief after each of her thrice-weekly TMJ and cervical spine manipulations for the first month. The patient was virtually pain-free after 12 treatments (one month) with no recurrence after three months. A recurrence two years later was relieved after four manipulations. Hruby (1985) reported two cases of patients with TMJ pain. The first case had no pain or discomfort after three visits with manipulation to the TMJ and spine. The second case experienced almost no discomfort two weeks after being treated with cranial and cervical manipulation.

Case reports (mobilization). Passero et al. (1985) describe two cases, each suffering from headache, and cervical and upper back pain. Dental exams revealed TMJ dysfunction and spasm of the pterygoid muscles. Each case was fitted with a flat-plane mandibular orthopedic appliance and underwent intensive physical therapy two to three times weekly for five to seven months. Physical therapy consisted of hot packs, high-voltage galvanism, ultrasound, trigger-point massage and injections with 2 percent lidocaine hydrochloride, spray and stretch, and intermittent cervical traction. Both patients' pain was subjectively eliminated or greatly diminished after their courses of care were completed.

In summary, the current literature is insufficient to either support or refute the use of cervical spine manipulation and/or mobilization for patients with TMJ disorders.

OTHER ENTITIES

Blood Pressure and Heart Rate

Four studies address the influence of cervical spine manipulation on blood pressure: one RCT (Vernon, 1986), and three cohort studies (McKnight and DeBoer, 1988; Christian et al., 1988; Nansel et al., 1991).

Randomized controlled trial. Vernon et al. (1986) conducted an RCT of 27 asymptomatic subjects: nine received one rotation manipulation, eight received a sham adjustment, and ten received nothing. There were no differences between groups with respect to blood pressure or heart rate from five to 40 minutes after the adjustment.

Other studies. McKnight and DeBoer (1988) conducted a cohort study of 75 asymptomatic subjects: 53 received one Gonstead cervical adjustment and 22 received palpation only. Statistically significant reductions in both systolic (mean decrease of 2.8 mm Hg) and diastolic (mean decrease of 2.6 mm Hg) blood pressures were found in the manipulated group ($P<0.01$) but not in the control group ($P>0.01$) within one minute of treatment. Fourteen (26.4 percent) of the manipulated subjects and none of the control subjects had more than a ten point decrease in blood pressure post treatment.

Christian et al. (1988) conducted a four-group study: (1) asymptomatic subjects who received spinal manipulative therapy (n=10); (2) subjects with cervical or thoracic pain who received SMT (spinal manual therapy) (n=10), (3) asymptomatic subjects who received a sham SMT (n=10), and (4) subjects with cervical or thoracic pain who received a sham SMT (n=10). No significant differences were found between groups at five and 30 minutes after treatment.

Nansel et al. (1991) reported the results of a cohort study in which 12 asymptomatic subjects with cervical lateral-flexion asymmetries received one Gonstead manipulation to the lower cervical spine and 12 similar subjects received a sham adjustment only. No significant differences were found between groups with respect to blood pressure or heart rate from five minutes to four hours after treatment.

In summary, the literature is too limited to make any determinations with respect to the effect of cervical spine manipulation on blood pressure and heart rate.

Cervical Spine/Intersegmental Motion

Three cohort studies and two case series were found in the literature that report the effect of cervical manipulation on cervical spine range of motion and/or intersegmental movement.

Cohort studies. Hviid (1971) conducted a cohort study of 227 subjects (127 patients and 100 subjects from the normal population). The patients were treated with five cervical rotary manipulations and range of motion assessed (unblinded) after each treatment. Eighty-four patients had an increase in rotation after one treatment and 72 maintained an increase from pretreatment to prior to the fifth treatment. Overall, there was a mean increase of 9 percent over pretreatment rotation. The normal population had 177.4 degrees of total rotation versus 171.6 degrees for the patients prior to their fifth treatment.

Nansel et al. (1989) conducted a four group cohort study of 43 subjects with left-right end range lateral-flexion asymmetries: nine subjects received no intervention, nine received a set-up but no thrust, 14 subjects received a Gonstead-type manipulation to the restricted side of the cervical spine (C5-T1), and 11 received manipulation to the least restricted side. Thirty to 45 minutes following treatment, mean asymmetries (as assessed by blind goniometric evaluation) were significantly reduced only in the manipulation groups, and to a much greater extent in the manipulation-to-the-most-restricted-side group ($P<0.001$). Nansel et al. (1990) completed another study of subjects with lateral flexion asymmetries, comparing 16 patients with previous neck trauma to 16 subjects with no trauma history. A Gonstead-type lower cervical manipulation (C6-T1) decreased mean asymmetries from 13.7 to 1.6 (30 minutes post-adjustment) to 3.8, 48 hours later in the no-previous-trauma group. In the previous trauma group, asymmetry improvement was not maintained (15.2 pre-adjustment to 2.7 30 minutes post-adjustment to 11.4, 48 hours later). Nansel et al. (1992) also compared the effect of upper and lower cervical Gonstead-type manipulations on correcting rotation and lateral flexion asymmetries. Upper cervical adjustments improved rotational asymmetries whereas lower cervical manipulations improved lateral flexion asymmetries, as assessed by blind goniometric evaluations within 30 minutes after adjustments.

Case series. Jirout (1985) described a case series of 200 patients with C2-C3 rotation restrictions who underwent one or two treatments of cervical manipulation and/or postisometric relaxation. All cases had their restrictions removed, 107 (53.5 percent) "felt better," 35 (17.5 percent) reported no symptoms, and 47 (23.5 percent) were lost to follow-up.

Yeomans (1992) used cervical stress radiography to assess the effect of chiropractic treatment on spinal mobility in 58 patients who were treated three times weekly for two to six weeks. Statistically significant improvements in spinal mobility were observed at each spinal level ($P<0.05$), except at C1.

In summary, the literature described above and in previous sections on Chronic Neck Pain and on Migraine Headache provides evidence that manipulation of the cervical spine increases range of motion and intersegmental mobility.

Cervical Spine Curvature

Two cohort studies and two case series addressed the influence of cervical spine manipulation on cervical lordosis. The relationship between either of these and improved patient functioning is not well established.

Cohort studies. Leach (1983) conducted a retrospective cohort study of 35 patients with cervical hypolordosis or kyphosis, of which 20 received chiropractic manipulation designed to affect curvature, 9 received a cervical pillow in addition to the manipulation, and 6 received a rotation manipulation (i.e., designed not to affect curvature). The mean change in cervical curve depth, as measured on X ray, was 4.55 in the first group ($P<0.01$), 2.22 in the second group ($P<0.05$), and –0.83 ($P>0.05$) in the third group. Data were not presented to calculate statistics to assess statistical significance between groups.

Pedersen (1990) conducted a cohort study of 26 patients, nine of whom had minor cervical trauma of less than two months' duration. After an average of 14 days in which the trauma patients received five chiropractic manipulations and the non-trauma patients received only noncervical treatment, significant changes occurred in cervical curve depths (as assessed by pre- and post-X rays) in both groups ($P<0.01$). It could not be concluded if there were significant differences between groups.

Case series. Jirout (1972) reported on a series of 250 subjects with segmental blockade of C4-C6 in lateroflexion who were treated with one supine cervical manipulation. Pre- and post-lateroflexion X rays were compared to assess changes in the projection of the spinous processes on vertebral bodies. In 197 (79 percent) of the cases, ventral tilting was increased in all segments of either the upper or lower cervical spine.

Plaugher et al. (1990) analyzed pre- and post-full-spine X rays of 49 patients who had an average of 6.5 Gonstead full-spine adjustments. No statistically significant changes were observed in cervical lordosis as measured on static X ray by an evaluator blind to pre-post status.

In summary, evidence from the literature is insufficient to support or refute the use of cervical spine manipulation for influencing cervical curvatures.

Miscellaneous

The effect of manipulation of the cervical spine on several other conditions or physiological states is addressed in many studies, primarily case series and case reports. These conditions include gastric tone (Wiles, 1980), muscle strength (Rebechini et al., 1981; Lowden et al., 1986; Bonci and Ratliff, 1990), torticollis (Hammond, 1983), bruxism (Nykoliation and Cassidy, 1984), cervical spondylolisthesis (Rowe and Steiman, 1987), Barre-Lieou (Bergmann and Porter, 1987), low-back pain (Hoiriis, 1989; Vaillancourt and Collins, 1993; Robinson et al., 1993), infantile colic (Klougart et al., 1989), otitis media (Hobbs and Rasmussen, 1991; Phillips, 1992), Tourette's Syndrome (Trotta, 1989), esophoria and other visual disturbances (Schutte et al., 1989; Gorman, 1993), tinnitus (Terrett, 1989), seizure disorders (Wing and Hargrave-Wilson, 1974; Goodman and Mosby, 1990; Duff, 1992), vertigo (Jirout, 1985; Droz, 1985; Bergmann and Porter, 1987; Fitz-Ritson, 1991), dizziness (Vernon, 1982a; Stodolny and Chmielewski, 1989; McConekey et al., 1990; Gorman, 1993), nausea (Livingston, 1968; Vernon, 1982a; Droz and Crot, 1985), cervical disc herniation (Siciliano et al., 1992), lumbar muscle tone (Nansel et al., 1993), and plasma levels of beta-endorphin (Vernon et al., 1986; Christian et al., 1988), ACTH and cortisol (Christian et al., 1988), and epinephrine, norepinephrine and dopamine (Nansel et al., 1991).

Insufficient evidence exists to support or refute the use of cervical spine mobilization or manipulation for any of the above entities.

COMPLICATIONS

Articles documenting more than 110 cases of complications allegedly arising from cervical spine manipulation have been published in English (see References on Treatment Complications, p. 109). The vast majority of these complications involved vertebrobasilar accidents (VBA) with consequences such as brainstem and/or cerebellar infarction, Wallenberg's Syndrome (obstruction of the posterior inferior cerebellar artery), and Locked-In Syndrome (occlusion of basilar artery). Other reported complications include spinal cord compression, vertebral fracture, tracheal rupture, diaphragm paralysis, internal carotid hematoma, and cardiac arrest.

Complications occurred in patients who had received manipulation uneventfully in the past, without obvious risk factors for cardiovascular accidents (CVAs) (e.g., arteriosclerosis, hypertension, heavy smoking, oral contraceptive use), without previous trauma, and with negative positional tests designed to assess vertebral artery sufficiency. It is apparent that the predisposing factors for CVAs in general are dissimilar to those for the post-manipulative vertebral artery dissections. However, in many cases, the manipulator failed to cease treatment even after signs and symptoms of vertebrobasilar ischemia (e.g., dizziness, vertigo, nausea, loss of consciousness). No complications were reported among the subjects who received cervical spine manipulation in the studies described in the efficacy section [p. 10].

The following discussion summarizes the complications resulting from cervical spine manipulation, according to presenting complaint. Table 5 and Table 6 present a listing of the case reports of complications of cervical spine manipulation, organized by type of complication, found in our literature search.

Neck pain. Thirty-seven case reports involved subjects complaining of neck pain or neck ache of durations ranging from one day to more than two years. Many patients complained of recurrent or chronic pain for many years. Chiropractors manipulated 25 (68 percent) of the subjects. Rotation manipulations were used in 10 of the 13 cases (77 percent) in which type of treatment was described. Twenty-two (60 percent) became symptomatic (e.g., showed signs or symptoms of a vertebrobasilar accident) after the first adjustment for their present complaint, and 25 (68 percent) had symptoms during or immediately following the adjustment.

Twenty-four subjects (65 percent) suffered from the consequences of vertebrobasilar ischemia (VBI). Eight developed Wallenberg's Syndrome, seven had brainstem and/or cerebellar infarctions, eight were diagnosed with VBA spasm, stenosis, or dissection, and one developed Locked-In Syndrome. Five of the 24 subjects died and nine (VBIs) were left with serious residual symptoms (e.g., paralysis, neurological deficit, or other permanent functional impairment). The other non-VBI subjects (13 of 37) developed complications from undiagnosed spinal cord tumors or infections, diaphragm paralysis, vertebral fractures, and internal carotid artery hematomas. Five of these subjects were left with serious residual symptoms.

Neck stiffness. Ten case reports involved subjects complaining of neck stiffness. Chiropractors manipulated seven (70 percent) of the subjects. Rotation manipulations were used in six of the eight cases (75 percent) in which type of treatment was described. Seven (70 percent) became symptomatic after the first adjustment for their present complaint, and an equal percentage had symptoms during or immediately following the adjustment.

Eight subjects (80 percent) suffered from the consequences of VBI. Four developed Wallenberg's Syndrome, three had brainstem infarctions, and one had a vertebral artery dissection. Two of these subjects died and four were left with serious residual symptoms. The other two subjects of the ten with neck stiffness (20 percent) devel-

Table 5

Characteristics of Complications from Cervical Spine Manipulations, According to Presenting Complaint

	Neck Pain (n=37)	Stiffness (n=10)	Head & Neck (n=17)	Headache (n=23)	Oth/Uk (n=31)
Subject Age, mean years	43.0	49.4	34.5	36.9	36.7
Subject Sex					
Male	25 (68)	4 (40)	9 (53)	12 (52)	13 (42)
Female	12 (32)	4 (40)	6 (35)	8 (35)	18 (58)
Unknown	0 (0)	2 (20)	2 (12)	3 (13)	0 (0)
Therapist					
Chiropractor	25 (68)	7 (70)	13 (76)	16 (70)	25 (81)
Osteopath	5 (13)	0 (0)	0 (0)	2 (9)	1 (3)
MD	2 (5)	0 (0)	1 (6)	1 (4)	1 (3)
Other/Unknown	5 (14)	3 (30)	3 (18)	4 (17)	4 (13)
Manipulation					
Rotation Included	10 (27)	6 (60)	6 (35)	14 (61)	9 (29)
Other Type	3 (8)	2 (20)	1 (6)	0 (0)	4 (13)
Unknown	24 (65)	2 (20)	10 (59)	9 (39)	18 (58)
First Symptoms					
During Therapy	6 (16)	0 (0)	3 (18)	5 (22)	1 (3)
Within Seconds	19 (52)	7 (70)	10 (59)	10 (43)	21 (68)
Within 24 Hours	6 (16)	3 (30)	3 (18)	7 (30)	7 (22)
Later	6 (16)	0 (0)	1 (6)	1 (5)	2 (7)
Diagnosis					
Wallenberg's Syndrome	8 (22)	4 (40)	1 (6)	6 (26)	4 (13)
Brain/Cerebellar Infarct	7 (19)	3 (30)	8 (47)	9 (39)	15 (48)
VBA Spasm/Dissection	8 (22)	1 (10)	3 (18)	5 (22)	1 (3)
Locked-In Syndrome	1 (3)	0 (0)	1 (6)	0 (0)	1 (3)
Other/Unknown	0 (0)	2 (20)	4 (23)	3 (13)	10 (32)
Outcome					
No/Minimal Impairment	16 (43)	2 (20)	2 (12)	10 (43)	12 (39)
Major Residual Symptoms	14 (38)	6 (60)		11 (65)	8 (35)
Death	5 (14)	2 (20)	4 (23)	5 (22)	5 (16)
Unknown	2 (5)	0 (0)	0 (0)	0 (0)	2 (6)

Note: *Percentages are in parentheses unless otherwise noted.

Table 6

Complications Resulting from Treatments of the Cervical Spine

Treatment	Complication	Incidence
Cervical spine manipulation[1]	VBA or other complication[2]	1.46/1,000,000 manipulations
	Major impairment[3]	6.39/10,000,000 manipulations
	Death	2.68/10,000,000 manipulations
Cervical spine surgery[4]	Neurologic complication[5]	15.6/1000 surgeries
	Death	6.9/1000 surgeries
Non-Steroidal Anti-Inflammatory Drugs (NSAIDS)[6]	Serious GI event[7]	3.2/1000 subjects (age 65+)
		0.39/1000 subjects (age <65)
		1/1000 subjects (all ages)
Naprosyn[8]	GI bleeding and/or perforation	<1/100 subjects
	Renal failure	<1/100 subjects
	Congestive heart failure	<1/100 subjects
Indocin[8]	Peptic ulcer	<1/100 subjects
	Toxic hepatitis	<1/100 subjects
	Coma	<1/100 subjects
	Congestive heart failure	<1/100 subjects
	Acute anaphylaxis	<1/100 subjects
	Renal failure	<1/100 subjects
Motrin[8]	Gastric or duodenal ulcer	<1/100 subjects
	GI bleeding and/or perforation	<1/100 subjects
	Hepatitis	<1/100 subjects
	Pancreatitis	<1/100 subjects
	Aseptic meningitis	<1/100 subjects
	Coma	<1/100 subjects
	Congestive heart failure	<1/100 subjects
	Anaphylaxis	<1/100 subjects
	Acute renal failure	<1/100 subjects

Table 6—continued

[1]Data from case reports; total cervical manipulations estimated from community-based study of chiropractic services (Shekelle and Brook, 1991)

[2]Other complications include spinal cord compression, vertebral fracture, tracheal rupture, diaphragm paralysis, internal carotid hematoma, and cardiac arrest

[3]Major impairments include paralysis, neurological deficit, or other permanent functional impairment

[4]Data from 1982-1987 surveys of the Cervical Spine Research Society; validity questionable because of unknown response rates and generalizability may be limited due to select group of surgeons

[5]Neurologic complications include spinal cord or nerve root injury, recurrent laryngeal nerve palsy, dural leak, and injury to cervical sympathetic (Horner's syndrome)

[6]Data from meta-analysis of gastrointestinal complications related to use of nonsteroidal anti-inflammatory drugs (Gabriel et al., 1991)

[7]Serious GI events include bleeding, perforation, or other adverse GI event resulting in hospitalization or death

[8]Data from *Physicians' Desk Reference;* selected complications based on reports in clinical trials, in the literature, and on voluntary reports since marketing

oped complications from extradural spinal cord compression and diaphragm paralysis, respectively, and were left with serious residual symptoms.

Head and neck pain/stiffness. Seventeen case reports involved subjects complaining of both head and neck pain or head pain and neck stiffness. Chiropractors manipulated 13 (76 percent) of the subjects. Rotation manipulations were used in six of the eight cases (75 percent) in which type of treatment was described. Eight (47 percent) became symptomatic after the first adjustment for their present complaint, and 13 (76 percent) had symptoms during or immediately following the adjustment.

Fifteen subjects (88 percent) suffered from the consequences of VBI. One developed Wallenberg's Syndrome, eight had brainstem infarctions, one had a cerebral infarction, three had vertebral artery subintimal tears, one developed Locked-In Syndrome, and one suffered an occipital lobe stroke. Four of these subjects died and 10 were left with serious residual symptoms. One of the other two subjects went into cardiac arrest during the adjustment, while the other had an adjustment that caused a fracture of C6 that left her with serious residual symptoms.

Headache. Twenty-three case reports involved subjects complaining of headache of durations ranging from four hours to 11 years. Chiropractors manipulated 16 (70 percent) of the subjects. Rotation manipulations were used in all 14 of the cases in which type of treatment was described. Fifteen (65 percent) became symptomatic after the first adjustment for their present complaint, and 15 (65 percent) had symptoms during or immediately following the adjustment.

Twenty-one subjects (91 percent) suffered from the consequences of VBI. Six developed Wallenberg's Syndrome, nine suffered brainstem and/or cerebellar infarctions, five were diagnosed with VBA spasm, stenosis, or dissection, and one had a pseudoaneurysm. Five of these subjects died and eight were left with serious residual symptoms. The other two subjects had brainstem strokes resulting from an undiagnosed brainstem lesion and C2 dislocation, respectively. These subjects improved and were not left with significant neurological deficits.

Other conditions. Eighteen case reports involved subjects complaining of other conditions, including torticollis (4), back pain (5), head colds or hay fever (4), and abdominal distension (1). Four other subjects were essentially asymptomatic. Chiropractors manipulated 17 (94 percent) of the subjects. Rotation manipulations were used in six of the nine (67 percent) cases in which type of treatment was described. Thirteen (72 percent) became symptomatic after the first adjustment for their present complaint, and 15 (83 percent) had symptoms during or immediately following the adjustment.

Twelve subjects (67 percent) suffered from the consequences of VBI. Three developed Wallenberg's Syndrome, nine suffered brainstem and/or cerebellar infarctions, and one had a thalamic infarction. Two of these subjects died and five were left with serious residual symptoms. The other six subjects had manipulations that resulted in vertebral dislocations, fractures, and/or hematomas, or had undiagnosed spinal cord tumors that were aggravated by the manipulation. One of these subjects died and one was left with significant neurological deficits.

Unknown presentation. The authors of 13 case reports did not describe the complaints for which the subjects sought manipulative treatment. Chiropractors manipulated eight (61.5 percent) of the subjects. Rotation manipulations were used in three of the four (75 percent) cases in which type of treatment was described. All subjects became symptomatic after the first adjustment for their present complaint, and eight (61.5 percent) had symptoms during or immediately following the adjustment.

Twelve of the subjects (92 percent) suffered from the consequences of VBI. One developed Wallenberg's Syndrome, six suffered brainstem and/or cerebellar infarctions, two had vertebral artery stenosis, one developed Locked-In Syndrome, and two cases were not reported. Two of these twelve subjects died and six were left with serious residual symptoms. The other subject recovered after his masseur allegedly ruptured his trachea.

In summary, of the 118 documented cases of complications from cervical spine manipulation described above, 92 involved vertebrobasilar (VBA) accidents. Twenty-one cases resulted in death, and 52 survived with serious neurological deficit, paralysis, or other permanent functional impairment. Terrett (1987) reported 26 deaths from 107 cases in English and non-English literature from 1934–1984, and 28 deaths from 113 cases described in the literature from 1934–1987 (Terrett, 1990).[2] Terrett's (1990) analysis revealed 21 deaths or cases with serious neurological sequelae that could have been prevented by the early recognition of VBA signs and symptoms.

Frequency. Because of the uncertainty of both caseload and the number of cervical manipulations that patients receive over a specified period of time, it is difficult to estimate the frequency of vertebrobasilar accidents and other complications among patients undergoing cervical spine manipulation. The risk of complications has been estimated to be between one in 40,000 manipulations for mild complications (Dvorak, 1985) and one in 400,000 to over one million manipulations for serious complications (Dvorak, 1985; Gutmann, 1983; Patijn, 1991). Dvorak (1991) reported no serious neurological complications during one year among 460 physicians and approximately 150,000 cervical manipulations.

In calculating a complication rate, we made an allowance for under-reporting. We have estimated under-reporting by a factor of 10 and although this figure is speculative, it does seem reasonable. At the very least, if many more people were having serious complications than are reported (under-reporting 100- or 1,000-fold), it is not reasonable that this would escape the attention of other providers involved in the care.

[2]Complete citations to the literature on treatment complications resulting from treatment of the cervical spine begin on p. 109. Unless otherwise noted, the references in this section pertain to that list of references.

Chiropractors perform about 90 percent of manipulation in the United States. Using data from a community-based study of the use of chiropractic services (Shekelle and Brook, 1991) to provide a rough estimate of the number of cervical spine manipulations delivered in the United States, and assuming that published case reports represent one-tenth of the actual complication caseload, the rate of vertebrobasilar accidents (VBA) or other complications (e.g., cord compression, fracture, hematoma, etc.) as a result of cervical spine manipulation is estimated to be 1.46 per one million manipulations. Using the same methodology, the rates of serious complications and death from cervical spine manipulation are estimated to be 6.39 per 10,000,000 manipulations and 2.68 per 10,000,000 manipulations, respectively. Table 6 (p. 36) shows the estimated incidence rates for complications as well as rates from other cervical spine treatments and drugs used to relieve cervical symptoms.

Systematic reports of complication rates are necessary to calculate a more precise estimate of risk. The true incidence of serious complications from cervical spine manipulation may be smaller and is probably modified by clinical presentation, appropriate history-taking and examination procedures, and the use of specific types of manual therapy.

Chapter Three

ANALYSIS OF THE APPROPRIATENESS RATINGS

For each indication for cervical or spinal manipulation or mobilization, the median was used to measure the central tendency of the nine panelists' ratings and the mean absolute distance from the median was used to measure the dispersion of the ratings. These measures are well suited, we believe, to the appropriateness scale.

Our 1 to 9 scale is an ordinal scale. It ranks excess of benefit over risk (including negative values when risks exceed benefit). A 9 is always more appropriate than an 8, and an 8 is always more appropriate than a 7. But risk-benefit levels are not specified for each point on the scale, so that a difference between a 9 and an 8 is not necessarily the same as the difference between an 8 and a 7. This scale characteristic suggests that we should avoid such measures as means and standard deviations that treat intervals as though they were equal.

Our scale does have some characteristics of an interval scale, however. The center of the scale (5) is well anchored at the point at which risk equals benefit. Although the ends (1 and 9) are not precisely specified, they are anchored to some degree. At 1, risks exceed benefits by a sufficiently wide margin that the procedure should definitely not be done. At 9, it definitely should be done.

It is established that using interval measures on ordinal scales seldom has much effect on the results. Shunning interval measures entirely would eliminate information. A four-point difference on our scale may not represent precisely four times as big a difference in the excess of benefit over risk as a one-point difference, but it certainly represents a bigger difference. A strictly ordinal measure would not distinguish between them.

Table 7 describes the average median, the mean absolute deviation from the median, and the percentage of agreement for the initial and final appropriateness ratings for spinal manipulation or mobilization for neck pain and headache. The table shows that the ratings changed from an initial median of 4.60 to a final median of 4.02. The table also shows a decrease in dispersion between the initial and final ratings.

On what portion of the indications did the panelists agree and disagree? Our preferred definition of agreement is that after discarding one extreme high and one extreme low rating, the remaining seven fall within any three-point range. According to our definition, at the conclusion of the process, panelists agreed on the ratings in 40 percent of the indications. Our preferred definition of disagreement is that, after

Table 7

Median Ratings and Extent of Agreement and Disagreement on Appropriateness Ratings for Spinal Manipulation or Mobilization

Item	Initial Rating	Final Ratings
Number of indications	1,171	1,436
Average median	4.60	4.02
Mean absolute deviation from median	1.51	1.14
Percentage of agreement	19.98%	39.97%
Percentage of disagreement	10.08%	2.09%

discarding one extreme high and one extreme low rating, at least two of the remaining seven fall in the lowest three-point region (1 to 3), and at least two fall in the highest. Table 7 shows that the panelists disagreed on the ratings in only 2 percent of the indications. For comparison, using the same definition for disagreement, a similar multidisciplinary panel of experts had disagreement on 3 percent of 1,550 indications for manipulation of the lumbar spine.[1]

We also classified indications into one of three categories of appropriateness: inappropriate, uncertain, or appropriate. We classified an indication as "uncertain" for either of two reasons: The benefits and risk of doing the procedure were considered roughly the same (a median rating of 4 to 6) or the panelists disagreed on the proper rating. An indication was called "appropriate" if the panelists assigned a median rating in the 7 to 9 range without disagreement, and it was "inappropriate" if they assigned a 1 to 3 rating without disagreement. Table 8 categorizes the final indications by their appropriateness ratings. Forty-three percent of indications were rated inappropriate. Appropriate and uncertain indications each accounted for 16 percent and 41 percent of the total.

Table 8

Categories of Appropriateness of 1,436 Indications for Cervical Manipulation and Mobilization

Category	Number of Indications	Percentage of Indications
Inappropriate	623	43%
Uncertain	586	41%
Appropriate	122	16%

[1]In previous publications on manipulation of the lumbar spine, the disagreement for the multidisciplinary panel was reported as 12 percent. The difference occurs because in past consensus panels (including both a full chiropractic panel and a mixed medical and chiropractic panel), RAND used a different definition of disagreements. The definition of disagreement was that, after disregarding one extreme high and one extreme low rating, at least one of the remaining seven fall in the lowest three-point region (1 to 3) and at least one falls in the highest. Under this definition, the multidisciplinary panel for manipulation and the lumbar spine disagreed on 12 percent of the indications. The cervical spine panel disagreed on 13.7 percent of the indications using this older definition.

The above analysis, however, represents aggregate values for both mobilization and manipulation. As seen in Tables 8–10, differences existed in the ratings of these two forms of therapy.

A comparison of Tables 8 and 9 shows that more indications were rated as inappropriate for manipulation than for mobilization and that the category of uncertain was largest for mobilization.

The level of disagreements also differed when manipulation and mobilization were considered independently. For mobilization, the panel disagreed on 0.9 percent of indications, whereas for manipulation, the panel disagreed on 3.3 percent of indications.

Comparing the results on manipulation of the two professions involved in the panel, chiropractic and medicine, the mean rating for appropriateness for the former is 4.51 and 2.62 for the latter. Furthermore, the mean rating of each medical physician was lower than that of any of the chiropractors. In the case of mobilization, the ratings were 5.01 for the chiropractors and 4.05 for the medical physicians. However, these results are less clear because one medical physician on the panel was more likely to rate mobilization appropriate than some of the chiropractors. The results do suggest that those using manual therapies—specifically, in this instance, chiropractors—are more likely to rate such therapies as appropriate than those who do not. This result has been shown to be the case with other panels, that is, those using the procedure are more likely to rate it as appropriate.

The low average median rating and the large number of indications rated inappropriate found in this study do not necessarily suggest that inappropriate care is being rendered. The case may be that in practice, manipulation or mobilization is used for highly appropriate indications. To understand the frequency of appropriate use of clinical spine mobilization and manipulation will require the collection of clinically

Table 9

Categories of Appropriateness of 736 Indications for Cervical Manipulation

Category	Number of Indications	Percentage of Indications
Inappropriate	424	57.6%
Uncertain	230	31.3%
Appropriate	82	11.1%
Total	736	100%

Table 10

Categories of Appropriateness of 700 Indications for Cervical Mobilization

Category	Number of Indications	Percentage of Indications
Inappropriate	199	28.4%
Uncertain	356	50.9%
Appropriate	145	20.7%
Total	700	100%

detailed patient level data on persons presenting with symptoms referable to the cervical spine.

The large number of responses that were indeterminant reflects that for the panel the risks and benefits were variably distributed for those indications. However, most of the indications with indeterminant levels of agreement were also judged to be of uncertain appropriateness (where risks and benefits were felt to be about equal or where there was insufficient information to tell). Most of the indications with panel disagreement also were given a medium rating of 4, 5, or 6. We interpret these results as indicating that much additional scientific data about the efficacy of cervical spine manipulation are needed.

INTERPRETING THE LISTINGS OF RESULTS

READING KEY

The final list of rated indications for spinal manipulation appears in Appendix B. Figure 4 provides a key to reading the results. Note that the indications represented in Figure 4 are for a patient with Chronic Intermittent Headache AND: No Clinical or Radiographic Risk Factors AND: Non-throbbing prodrome AND: cervical signs and/or symptoms AND: No c-spine radiographs and absence of clinical risk factors for manipulation AND: no prior SMT. In this case, the median rating for mobilization was 6, and, for manipulation, 5. However, the dispersion was greater for manipulation than for mobilization (1.2 versus 2.0 mean absolute deviation).

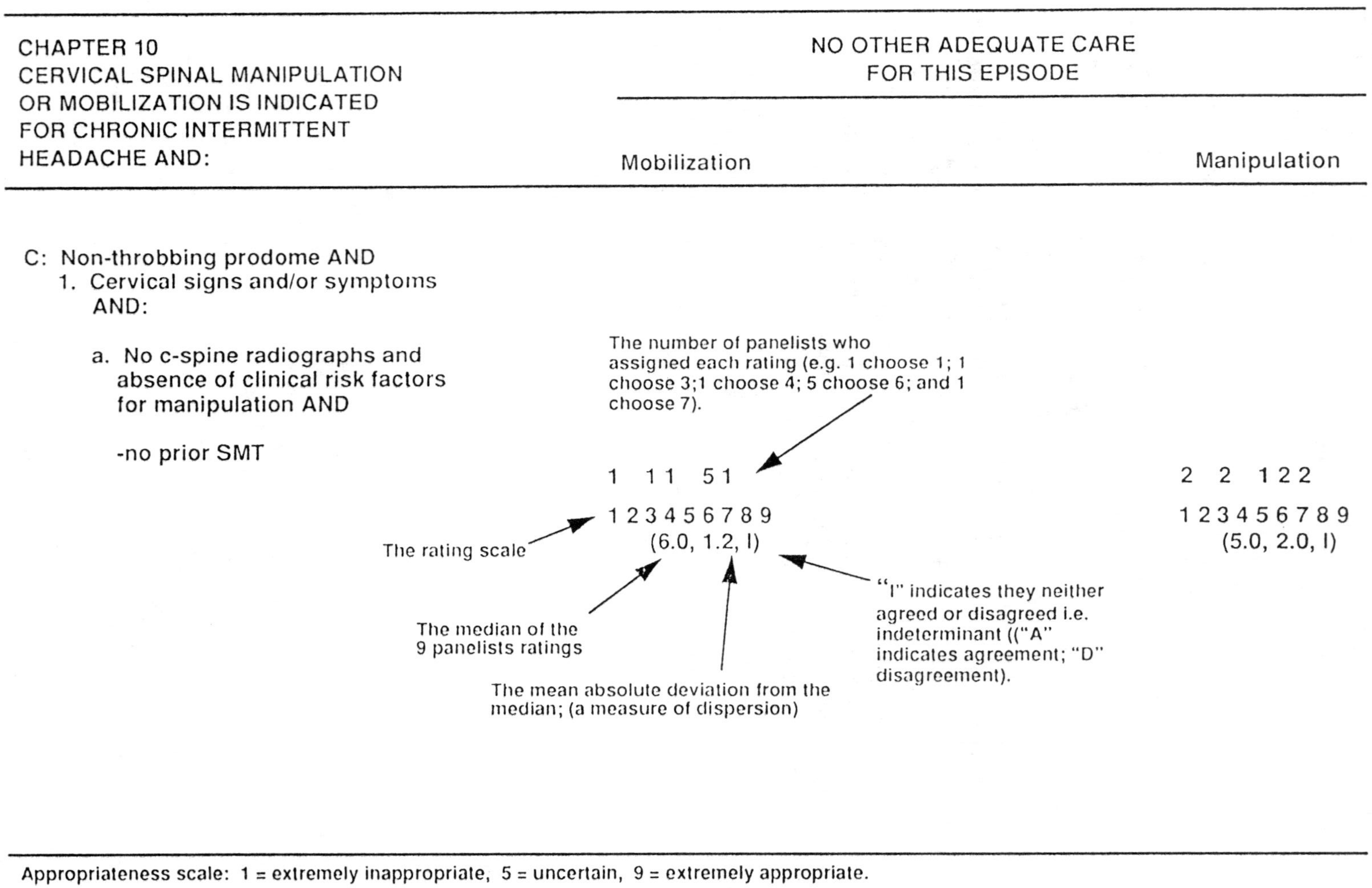

Figure 4—A Key to Reading the Final Results of Appropriateness Ratings for Each Indication for Cervical Manipulation and Mobilization

DEFINITIONS

Active range of motion
Extent of mobility attained by the patient without assistance.

Acute headache
Onset less than three weeks ago.

Acute neck pain
Pain or condition present less than three weeks (includes acute episodes of an intermittent condition).

Adequate course of conservative (nonsurgical, nonmanipulative) care
A trial of care of sufficient intensity and duration to normally achieve a favorable response.

Advanced imaging tests
Includes any of the following: CT, contrast CT, MRI, contrast MRI, or myelography.

Articular hypermobility
Treatment at the hypermobile joint.

Cervical manipulation
A controlled, judiciously applied dynamic thrust (adjustment) that may include combined extension and rotation of the upper cervical spinal segments, of high- or low-velocity and low-amplitude force directed to spinal joint segment within patient tolerance. Procedures often take joints into the "paraphysiological" space resulting in joint cavitation.

Cervical manipulation without combined extension and rotation
A controlled, judiciously applied dynamic thrust (adjustment), using pre-stress that minimizes hyperextension and rotation of the upper cervical spinal segments, of high- or low-velocity and low-amplitude force directed to spinal joint segments within patient tolerance. Procedures often take joints into the "paraphysiological" space resulting in joint cavitation.

Cervical mobilization
A controlled, judiciously applied force of low velocity and variable amplitude directed to spinal joint segment(s). Procedures usually do not take joints beyond the passive range of motion and do not result in joint cavitation.

Cervical radiographs
Standard orthogonal series of plain film radiographs.

Cervical signs or symptoms
Clinical findings to suggest cervical spine involvement: neck pain, myofascial trigger points, headache provoked by mechanical stress to cervical tissues or joint dysfunction.

Cervical SMT (Spinal Manual Therapy)
Spinal Manual Therapy is a generic label for a family of procedures that includes cervical manipulation and mobilization.

Chronic headache
Onset more than three months ago.

Chronic neck pain
Pain or condition present for more than three months.

Clinical risk factors for manipulation of the cervical spine without X rays
Patient over age 65, fever greater than 100 degrees F; prolonged corticosteroid use; unexplained weight loss; history of cancer; history of serious systemic inflammatory arthritides or vasculitides; endocrinopathies that affect calcium metabolism.

Clotting or bleeding tests
Clinical laboratory studies that measure the integrity of the coagulation process (i.e., prothrombin time, bleeding time, etc.).

Constant headache
Patient has had no pain-free periods since onset.

Definite radiculopathy
Symptoms, signs, or tests classical for radiculopathy, including any one of the following: unequivocal motor weakness or EMG changes; unequivocal asymmetric depressed reflexes; dermatomal hypalgesia; each of which is typically preceded or accompanied by radicular pain.

Electrodiagnostic tests
Includes tests of neurologic function (e.g., nerve conduction velocity, electromyography, somato sensory evoked potentials), but excluding surface electromyography.

Favorable response to prior SMT
Patient has received SMT to the neck for a similar complaint and experienced clinical benefit.

Headache
Complaint of pain in the head excluding the lower half of the face.

Herniated disc
Herniation of the intervertebral nucleus pulposus at any level in the cervical spine. Does not include disc bulge without herniation or small contained herniation with no evidence of nerve root impingement.

Imaging study shows no abnormality
Advanced imaging study shows no herniated disc, spinal foraminal osteophytosis, or central spinal stenosis.

Intermittent headache
Patient has had pain-free periods since onset.

Joint dysfunction
Decreased or aberrant segmental or regional joint mobility excluding hypermobility but including tender or hypertonic contraction of the paraspinal muscles.

Local pathology
A mechanical or physiologic lesion external to the spine that is the source of symptoms and signs.

Major neurologic findings
At least one of the following: neurologic signs of cervical myelopathy; progressive unilateral muscle weakness and/or motor loss documented by repeat exam over time; sensory deficits other than those related to dermatomes or peripheral nerves.

Mild post-traumatic neurologic symptoms
Symptoms such as occipital headache, light headedness, concentration difficulties, sleep disturbances, loss of visual accommodation, with a normal neurological examination.

Minimally traumatic etiology
A history of trauma relatable to a patient's complaint, with no or minor negative implications.

Neck pain
Pain in the region of the cervical spine including the occipita-cervico and cervico-thoraco junctions.

No or unfavorable response to prior SMT
Patient has received SMT to the neck for a similar complaint and experienced equivocal or no clinical benefit.

No prior SMT
The patient has never received SMT to the neck for a similar complaint.

No radiculopathy
Absence of signs or symptoms that are listed in possible or definite radiculopathy.

Nontraumatic etiology
No history of trauma consistent with patient's complaint.

Pain of musculotendinous distribution
Pain consistent with anatomy of specific muscles and/or their attachments.

Passive range of motion
Extent of mobility attained with minimal effort by the patient and with clinician assistance.

Possible radiculopathy
Symptoms, signs, or tests suggestive of radiculopathy, including at least one of the following: sensory changes including paresthesia and/or hyperesthesia of a dermatomal distribution; pain radiation into the upper extremity that follows a dermatomal pattern; in the absence of symptoms, signs or tests of definite radiculopathy.

Prodrome
History of visual disturbances, dizziness, unilateral paresthesias, or mood changes associated with headache.

Provocative testing
Those tests or procedures that are performed to elicit physical or physiological expressions of vertebrobasilar insufficiency.

Psychosocial stress
Diagnosed depression; alcohol or narcotic dependence; recent suicide attempt; diagnosed severe anxiety. Evidence of stressful life situation such as bereavement, job change, job or family dissatisfaction.

Radiographic contraindications to manipulation of the cervical spine
Include, but are not limited to neoplastic disease in the cervical region; certain bone diseases including infections (e.g., discites, osteomyelitis, tuberculosis), Paget's disease, or severe osteoporosis; active inflammatory arthritis (ankylosing spondylitis, rheumatoid arthritis); septic arthritis; acute or unhealed fracture; obvious misalignment (of greater than 3 mm of translation, or greater than 11 percent of kyphotic angulation); some congenital anomalies such as unstable os odontoideum; ossification of the posterior longitudinal ligament; anterior-posterior spinal canal stenosis of less than or equal to 11 millimeters.

Radiographic findings of degenerative changes in the cervical spine
(a) *early*—minimal loss of disc height, minimal sclerosis, no visible osteophytes, no visible intervertebral foraminal encroachment;
(b) *moderate*—mild loss of disc height, mild sclerosis, small osteophytes, minimal intervertebral foraminal encroachment;
(c) *advanced*—multi-level significant loss of disc height, severe sclerosis, large osteophytes, severe intervertebral foraminal encroachment, probable canal/lateral stenosis.

Related cervical spine trauma
A history of trauma relatable to patient's complaint.

Spinal foraminal osteophytosis
Stenosis of greater than 50 percent or with evidence of nerve root impingement.

Spinal stenosis
Central spinal canal stenosis with anterior-posterior diameter of less than or equal to 11 millimeters.

Subacute headache
Onset between three weeks and three months.

Subacute neck pain
Pain or condition present for more than three weeks but less than three months.

Substantial traumatic etiology
A history of trauma relatable to a patient's complaint with more than minor negative implications. Average "fender bender" type automobile accident not considered substantial trauma.

Throbbing headache
Headache described as pulsing (quickly varying in intensity).

TMJ
Temporomandibular joint.

Appendix B

PANEL RATINGS OF INDICATIONS BY CHAPTER

- 1 - Mon Sep 25 12:29:24 1995

Chapter 1 CERVICAL SPINAL MANIPULATION OR MOBILIZATION IS APPROPRIATE WITH: ACUTE NECK PAIN AND SIGNS OF PAINFUL AND/OR LIMITED ACTIVE RANGE OF MOTION AND PAIN ANATOMICALLY CONSISTENT WITH A MUSCULOTENDINOUS DISTRIBUTION AND NO RADICULOPATHY AND	NO PRIOR SMT		FAVORABLE RESPONSE TO PRIOR SMT		NO RESPONSE TO PRIOR SMT		UNFAVORABLE RESPONSE TO PRIOR SMT		
	Mobilization	Manipulation	Mobilization	Manipulation	Mobilization	Manipulation	Mobilization	Manipulation	
A. Non-traumatic or minimally traumatic etiology AND									
1. No clinical risk factors for radiographic contraindications to cervical manipulation, and no cervical radiographs	3 6 1 2 3 4 5 6 7 8 9 (8.0, 0.7, I)	1 1 2 4 1 1 2 3 4 5 6 7 8 9 (8.0, 1.2, A)	1 1 4 3 1 2 3 4 5 6 7 8 9 (8.0, 0.7, A)	2 1 1 5 1 2 3 4 5 6 7 8 9 (9.0, 1.2, A)	2 3 1 2 1 1 2 3 4 5 6 7 8 9 (6.0, 1.1, I)	2 1 1 1 3 1 1 2 3 4 5 6 7 8 9 (6.0, 1.7, I)	1 2 1 4 1 1 2 3 4 5 6 7 8 9 (6.0, 1.1, A)	1 1 2 3 2 1 2 3 4 5 6 7 8 9 (4.0, 1.2, I)	(1- 8)
2. Presence of clinical risk factors for radiographic contraindications to cervical manipulation, and no cervical radiographs	2 1 4 2 1 2 3 4 5 6 7 8 9 (6.0, 1.2, I)	1 2 3 1 1 1 1 2 3 4 5 6 7 8 9 (3.0, 1.4, I)	1 1 1 5 1 1 2 3 4 5 6 7 8 9 (7.0, 0.9, I)	1 2 1 3 1 1 1 2 3 4 5 6 7 8 9 (5.0, 1.9, I)	1 1 1 2 4 1 2 3 4 5 6 7 8 9 (5.0, 1.1, A)	1 3 2 1 2 1 2 3 4 5 6 7 8 9 (3.0, 1.3, I)	1 1 4 2 1 1 2 3 4 5 6 7 8 9 (3.0, 0.8, I)	5 3 1 1 2 3 4 5 6 7 8 9 (1.0, 0.7, A)	(9- 16)
3. Cervical radiographs show no contraindications to cervical manipulation	1 1 5 2 1 2 3 4 5 6 7 8 9 (8.0, 0.6, A)	1 1 1 3 3 1 2 3 4 5 6 7 8 9 (8.0, 1.3, A)	1 5 3 1 2 3 4 5 6 7 8 9 (8.0, 0.4, A)	1 2 6 1 2 3 4 5 6 7 8 9 (9.0, 1.0, A)	1 1 3 2 1 1 1 2 3 4 5 6 7 8 9 (6.0, 1.2, I)	1 1 1 1 3 1 1 1 2 3 4 5 6 7 8 9 (7.0, 1.7, I)	1 1 3 4 1 2 3 4 5 6 7 8 9 (5.0, 0.9, A)	1 2 1 2 3 1 2 3 4 5 6 7 8 9 (5.0, 1.3, I)	(17- 24)
B. Clinically substantial traumatic etiology AND									
1. No clinical risk factors for radiographic contraindications to cervical manipulation, and no cervical radiographs	1 1 2 1 3 1 1 2 3 4 5 6 7 8 9 (5.0, 1.6, I)	3 2 2 1 1 1 2 3 4 5 6 7 8 9 (2.0, 1.3, A)	1 1 2 1 2 1 1 1 2 3 4 5 6 7 8 9 (5.0, 1.7, I)	3 3 1 1 1 1 2 3 4 5 6 7 8 9 (2.0, 1.8, I)	1 3 1 1 2 1 1 2 3 4 5 6 7 8 9 (3.0, 1.9, I)	2 3 1 2 1 1 2 3 4 5 6 7 8 9 (2.0, 1.4, I)	5 2 1 1 1 2 3 4 5 6 7 8 9 (1.0, 1.0, A)	6 2 1 1 2 3 4 5 6 7 8 9 (1.0, 0.6, A)	(25- 32)
2. Presence of clinical risk factors for radiographic contraindications to cervical manipulation, and no cervical radiographs	4 1 2 1 1 1 2 3 4 5 6 7 8 9 (2.0, 1.4, A)	5 3 1 1 2 3 4 5 6 7 8 9 (1.0, 0.7, A)	4 2 1 2 1 2 3 4 5 6 7 8 9 (3.0, 1.4, I)	5 1 1 2 1 2 3 4 5 6 7 8 9 (1.0, 1.0, A)	3 3 1 2 1 2 3 4 5 6 7 8 9 (2.0, 1.3, A)	7 1 1 1 2 3 4 5 6 7 8 9 (1.0, 0.4, A)	7 1 1 1 2 3 4 5 6 7 8 9 (1.0, 0.6, A)	9 1 2 3 4 5 6 7 8 9 (1.0, 0.0, A)	(33- 40)
3. Cervical radiographs show no contraindications to cervical manipulation	1 6 2 1 2 3 4 5 6 7 8 9 (7.0, 0.3, A)	3 2 3 1 1 2 3 4 5 6 7 8 9 (6.0, 0.9, I)	2 2 5 1 2 3 4 5 6 7 8 9 (8.0, 0.7, A)	1 1 2 2 2 1 1 2 3 4 5 6 7 8 9 (7.0, 1.2, I)	1 3 2 3 1 2 3 4 5 6 7 8 9 (6.0, 1.0, I)	2 2 4 1 1 2 3 4 5 6 7 8 9 (6.0, 1.0, I)	1 2 2 3 1 1 2 3 4 5 6 7 8 9 (4.0, 1.0, I)	2 3 2 2 1 2 3 4 5 6 7 8 9 (3.0, 1.1, I)	(41- 48)

Appropriateness scale: 1 = extremely inappropriate, 5 = uncertain, 9 = extremely appropriate.

```
Chapter 2
CERVICAL SPINAL MANIPULATION OR MOBILIZATION
IS APPROPRIATE WITH:
SUBACUTE OR CHRONIC NECK PAIN AND SIGNS OF
PAINFUL AND/OR LIMITED ACTIVE RANGE OF MOTION   NO OTHER ADEQUATE CONSERVATIVE       NONMANIPULATIVE CONSERVATIVE CARE
AND PAIN ANATOMICALLY CONSISTENT WITH A            CARE FOR THIS EPISODE              FOR THIS EPISODE HAS FAILED
MUSCULOTENDINOUS DISTRIBUTION AND              -----------------------------------  -----------------------------------
NO RADICULOPATHY AND                              Mobilization       Manipulation      Mobilization       Manipulation

CONTINUED PSYCHOSOCIAL STRESS AND

A. Non-traumatic or minimally traumatic
   etiology and no prior experience with SMT
   AND

   1. No clinical risk factors for
      radiographic contraindications to
      cervical manipulation, and no cervical        1     5 3   2       1 2 4       1       5 3   2       1 2 4
      radiographs                             1 2 3 4 5 6 7 8 9 1 2 3 4 5 6 7 8 9 1 2 3 4 5 6 7 8 9 1 2 3 4 5 6 7 8 9     (  1-  4)
                                                (7.0, 0.7, A)     (6.0, 1.7, I)     (7.0, 0.8, A)     (6.0, 1.7, I)
   2. Presence of clinical risk factors for
      radiographic contraindications to
      cervical manipulation, and no cervical  1 1 1   2 2 2     2 4   1 2         1 1 1 1   3 2     2 4 1 1   1
      radiographs                             1 2 3 4 5 6 7 8 9 1 2 3 4 5 6 7 8 9 1 2 3 4 5 6 7 8 9 1 2 3 4 5 6 7 8 9     (  5-  8)
                                                (5.0, 1.7, I)     (2.0, 1.1, I)     (6.0, 1.8, I)     (2.0, 1.0, A)
   3. Cervical radiographs show no
      contraindications to cervical                       2 6 1         1 1 2 4 1             1 5 3         1 1 1 2 4
      manipulation                            1 2 3 4 5 6 7 8 9 1 2 3 4 5 6 7 8 9 1 2 3 4 5 6 7 8 9 1 2 3 4 5 6 7 8 9     (  9- 12)
                                                (8.0, 0.3, A)     (8.0, 0.9, A)     (8.0, 0.4, A)     (8.0, 1.1, A)
B. Non-traumatic or minimally traumatic
   etiology and favorable prior experience
   with SMT AND

   1. No clinical risk factors for
      radiographic contraindications to
      cervical manipulation, and no cervical            1 4 4           2 1 2 4             1 3 4 1         2 1   5 1
      radiographs                             1 2 3 4 5 6 7 8 9 1 2 3 4 5 6 7 8 9 1 2 3 4 5 6 7 8 9 1 2 3 4 5 6 7 8 9     ( 13- 16)
                                                (7.0, 0.6, A)     (7.0, 1.0, I)     (8.0, 0.7, A)     (8.0, 1.0, I)
   2. Presence of clinical risk factors for
      radiographic contraindications to
      cervical manipulation, and no cervical      1 2 1 4 1     1 3 2 2   1               3   4 1 1     1 2 3 2   1
      radiographs                             1 2 3 4 5 6 7 8 9 1 2 3 4 5 6 7 8 9 1 2 3 4 5 6 7 8 9 1 2 3 4 5 6 7 8 9     ( 17- 20)
                                                (6.0, 1.0, A)     (3.0, 1.1, I)     (6.0, 1.0, A)     (3.0, 1.0, I)
   3. Cervical radiographs show no
      contraindications to cervical                       2 5 2           2 1 4 2             3 3 3           1 2 2 4
      manipulation                            1 2 3 4 5 6 7 8 9 1 2 3 4 5 6 7 8 9 1 2 3 4 5 6 7 8 9 1 2 3 4 5 6 7 8 9     ( 21- 24)
                                                (8.0, 0.4, A)     (8.0, 0.8, A)     (8.0, 0.7, A)     (8.0, 0.9, A)
```

Appropriateness scale: 1 = extremely inappropriate, 5 = uncertain, 9 = extremely appropriate.

```
Chapter 2
CERVICAL SPINAL MANIPULATION OR MOBILIZATION
IS APPROPRIATE WITH:
SUBACUTE OR CHRONIC NECK PAIN AND SIGNS OF
PAINFUL AND/OR LIMITED ACTIVE RANGE OF MOTION   NO OTHER ADEQUATE CONSERVATIVE        NONMANIPULATIVE CONSERVATIVE CARE
AND PAIN ANATOMICALLY CONSISTENT WITH A             CARE FOR THIS EPISODE                FOR THIS EPISODE HAS FAILED
MUSCULOTENDINOUS DISTRIBUTION AND               ------------------------------------  ------------------------------------
NO RADICULOPATHY AND                             Mobilization       Manipulation       Mobilization       Manipulation

CONTINUED PSYCHOSOCIAL STRESS AND

C. Non-traumatic or minimally traumatic
   etiology and no response to
   prior experience with SMT AND

   1. No clinical risk factors for
      radiographic contraindications to
      cervical manipulation, and no cervical          4 4 1      2   2 2 3              1   4 1 3      2 2     3 2
      radiographs                               1 2 3 4 5 6 7 8 9  1 2 3 4 5 6 7 8 9  1 2 3 4 5 6 7 8 9  1 2 3 4 5 6 7 8 9      ( 25- 28)
                                                  (7.0, 0.6, I)      (5.0, 1.2, A)      (6.0, 1.0, I)      (6.0, 1.8, I)
   2. Presence of clinical risk factors for
      radiographic contraindications to
      cervical manipulation, and no cervical        4 1 2 1 1        3 2 3   1                4 1 2   1 1  3 2 1 1 1 1
      radiographs                               1 2 3 4 5 6 7 8 9  1 2 3 4 5 6 7 8 9  1 2 3 4 5 6 7 8 9  1 2 3 4 5 6 7 8 9      ( 29- 32)
                                                  (4.0, 1.2, I)      (2.0, 1.0, A)      (4.0, 1.4, I)      (2.0, 1.4, I)
   3. Cervical radiographs show no
      contraindications to cervical                         3 6              2 3 1 3              1 2 4 2          3 1 2 1 2
      manipulation                              1 2 3 4 5 6 7 8 9  1 2 3 4 5 6 7 8 9  1 2 3 4 5 6 7 8 9  1 2 3 4 5 6 7 8 9      ( 33- 36)
                                                  (8.0, 0.3, A)      (6.0, 1.0, I)      (8.0, 0.7, A)      (7.0, 1.3, I)
D. Non-traumatic or minimally traumatic
   etiology and unfavorable response to
   prior experience with SMT AND

   1. No clinical risk factors for
      radiographic contraindications to
      cervical manipulation, and no cervical        1 1 3 4          1 2 3 2 1              2 1 1 4 1      2 2 1 1 2 1
      radiographs                               1 2 3 4 5 6 7 8 9  1 2 3 4 5 6 7 8 9  1 2 3 4 5 6 7 8 9  1 2 3 4 5 6 7 8 9      ( 37- 40)
                                                  (5.0, 0.8, A)      (3.0, 0.9, I)      (6.0, 1.1, I)      (3.0, 1.6, I)
   2. Presence of clinical risk factors for
      radiographic contraindications to
      cervical manipulation, and no cervical    1 3 3   2          8     1              3 4   1 1        7 1     1
      radiographs                               1 2 3 4 5 6 7 8 9  1 2 3 4 5 6 7 8 9  1 2 3 4 5 6 7 8 9  1 2 3 4 5 6 7 8 9      ( 41- 44)
                                                  (3.0, 1.0, A)      (1.0, 0.3, A)      (3.0, 0.9, A)      (1.0, 0.6, A)
   3. Cervical radiographs show no
      contraindications to cervical                   1 2 1 4 1    1   1   4   3              1 2 1 3 2    1   1   3 2 1 1
      manipulation                              1 2 3 4 5 6 7 8 9  1 2 3 4 5 6 7 8 9  1 2 3 4 5 6 7 8 9  1 2 3 4 5 6 7 8 9      ( 45- 48)
                                                  (7.0, 1.0, I)      (5.0, 1.3, I)      (7.0, 1.1, I)      (5.0, 1.4, I)
```

Appropriateness scale: 1 = extremely inappropriate, 5 = uncertain, 9 = extremely appropriate.

```
Chapter 2
CERVICAL SPINAL MANIPULATION OR MOBILIZATION
IS APPROPRIATE WITH:
SUBACUTE OR CHRONIC NECK PAIN AND SIGNS OF
PAINFUL AND/OR LIMITED ACTIVE RANGE OF MOTION   NO OTHER ADEQUATE CONSERVATIVE      NONMANIPULATIVE CONSERVATIVE CARE
AND PAIN ANATOMICALLY CONSISTENT WITH A           CARE FOR THIS EPISODE             FOR THIS EPISODE HAS FAILED
MUSCULOTENDINOUS DISTRIBUTION AND              ----------------------------------  ----------------------------------
NO RADICULOPATHY AND                             Mobilization       Manipulation     Mobilization       Manipulation

CONTINUED PSYCHOSOCIAL STRESS AND

E. Clinically substantial traumatic etiology
   and no prior experience with SMT AND

   1. No clinical risk factors for
      radiographic contraindications to
      cervical manipulation, and no cervical   2 1 2   3   1      3 3 2 1            2 1 1 2 1 1 1      3 2 2 2
      radiographs                              1 2 3 4 5 6 7 8 9  1 2 3 4 5 6 7 8 9  1 2 3 4 5 6 7 8 9  1 2 3 4 5 6 7 8 9   ( 49- 52)
                                                 (3.0, 1.7, I)      (2.0, 0.8, A)      (4.0, 1.7, I)      (2.0, 1.0, A)
   2. Presence of clinical risk factors for
      radiographic contraindications to
      cervical manipulation, and no cervical   2 6       1        5 4                2 5 1     1        6 3
      radiographs                              1 2 3 4 5 6 7 8 9  1 2 3 4 5 6 7 8 9  1 2 3 4 5 6 7 8 9  1 2 3 4 5 6 7 8 9   ( 53- 56)
                                                 (2.0, 0.7, A)      (1.0, 0.4, A)      (2.0, 0.8, A)      (1.0, 0.3, A)
   3. Cervical radiographs show no
      contraindications to cervical                      1 7 1            2 3 4                1 7 1            2 2 2 1 2
      manipulation                             1 2 3 4 5 6 7 8 9  1 2 3 4 5 6 7 8 9  1 2 3 4 5 6 7 8 9  1 2 3 4 5 6 7 8 9   ( 57- 60)
                                                 (7.0, 0.2, A)      (6.0, 0.7, I)      (7.0, 0.2, A)      (7.0, 1.2, I)
F. Clinically substantial traumatic etiology
   and favorable prior experience with SMT
   AND

   1. No clinical risk factors for
      radiographic contraindications to
      cervical manipulation, and no cervical   1   2 1 3   2      3 2 2 1 1          1   2 3 1 1 1      4 1 3   1
      radiographs                              1 2 3 4 5 6 7 8 9  1 2 3 4 5 6 7 8 9  1 2 3 4 5 6 7 8 9  1 2 3 4 5 6 7 8 9   ( 61- 64)
                                                 (5.0, 1.4, I)      (2.0, 1.1, A)      (4.0, 1.2, I)      (2.0, 1.1, A)
   2. Presence of clinical risk factors for
      radiographic contraindications to
      cervical manipulation, and no cervical   2 4 2     1        5 3 1              2 2 4     1        5 4
      radiographs                              1 2 3 4 5 6 7 8 9  1 2 3 4 5 6 7 8 9  1 2 3 4 5 6 7 8 9  1 2 3 4 5 6 7 8 9   ( 65- 68)
                                                 (2.0, 0.9, A)      (1.0, 0.6, A)      (3.0, 1.0, A)      (1.0, 0.4, A)
   3. Cervical radiographs show no
      contraindications to cervical                    1 3 3 2      1     1 3 1 3                2 5 1 1    1     3 1 1 1 2
      manipulation                             1 2 3 4 5 6 7 8 9  1 2 3 4 5 6 7 8 9  1 2 3 4 5 6 7 8 9  1 2 3 4 5 6 7 8 9   ( 69- 72)
                                                 (7.0, 0.8, I)      (6.0, 1.3, I)      (7.0, 0.6, A)      (6.0, 1.8, I)
```

Appropriateness scale: 1 = extremely inappropriate, 5 = uncertain, 9 = extremely appropriate.

```
Chapter 2
CERVICAL SPINAL MANIPULATION OR MOBILIZATION
IS APPROPRIATE WITH:
SUBACUTE OR CHRONIC NECK PAIN AND SIGNS OF
PAINFUL AND/OR LIMITED ACTIVE RANGE OF MOTION    NO OTHER ADEQUATE CONSERVATIVE       NONMANIPULATIVE CONSERVATIVE CARE
AND PAIN ANATOMICALLY CONSISTENT WITH A             CARE FOR THIS EPISODE              FOR THIS EPISODE HAS FAILED
MUSCULOTENDINOUS DISTRIBUTION AND               ---------------------------------- ----------------------------------
NO RADICULOPATHY AND                              Mobilization      Manipulation      Mobilization      Manipulation
---------------------------------------------------------------------------------------------------------------------------
CONTINUED PSYCHOSOCIAL STRESS AND

G. Clinically substantial traumatic etiology
   and no response to prior
   experience with SMT AND

   1. No clinical risk factors for
      radiographic contraindications to
      cervical manipulation, and no cervical   2 1 4 1   1         3 2 4             2 1 1 3 1 1       3 2 4
      radiographs                              1 2 3 4 5 6 7 8 9 1 2 3 4 5 6 7 8 9 1 2 3 4 5 6 7 8 9 1 2 3 4 5 6 7 8 9   ( 73- 76)
                                                 (3.0, 1.0, A)     (2.0, 0.8, A)     (4.0, 1.3, I)     (2.0, 0.8, A)
   2. Presence of clinical risk factors for
      radiographic contraindications to
      cervical manipulation, and no cervical   5 3       1         5 4               3 5       1       6 3
      radiographs                              1 2 3 4 5 6 7 8 9 1 2 3 4 5 6 7 8 9 1 2 3 4 5 6 7 8 9 1 2 3 4 5 6 7 8 9   ( 77- 80)
                                                 (1.0, 0.9, A)     (1.0, 0.4, A)     (2.0, 0.8, A)     (1.0, 0.3, A)
   3. Cervical radiographs show no
      contraindications to cervical                    3 2 3 1     1     1 3 3 1             2 1 1 4 1   1 1 1 1 1 3 1
      manipulation                             1 2 3 4 5 6 7 8 9 1 2 3 4 5 6 7 8 9 1 2 3 4 5 6 7 8 9 1 2 3 4 5 6 7 8 9   ( 81- 84)
                                                 (6.0, 0.9, I)     (5.0, 1.1, A)     (7.0, 1.1, I)     (6.0, 1.7, I)
H. Clinically substantial traumatic etiology
   and unfavorable response to prior
   experience with SMT AND

   1. No clinical risk factors for
      radiographic contraindications to
      cervical manipulation, and no cervical   3 4 2             6 3               3 4 2             8 1
      radiographs                              1 2 3 4 5 6 7 8 9 1 2 3 4 5 6 7 8 9 1 2 3 4 5 6 7 8 9 1 2 3 4 5 6 7 8 9   ( 85- 88)
                                                 (2.0, 0.6, A)     (1.0, 0.3, A)     (2.0, 0.6, A)     (1.0, 0.1, A)
   2. Presence of clinical risk factors for
      radiographic contraindications to
      cervical manipulation, and no cervical   8 1               9                 8 1               9
      radiographs                              1 2 3 4 5 6 7 8 9 1 2 3 4 5 6 7 8 9 1 2 3 4 5 6 7 8 9 1 2 3 4 5 6 7 8 9   ( 89- 92)
                                                 (1.0, 0.1, A)     (1.0, 0.0, A)     (1.0, 0.1, A)     (1.0, 0.0, A)
   3. Cervical radiographs show no
      contraindications to cervical                1 3 2 1 2       2 1 2   4           1 1 1 2 2 2     1 3     1 3 1
      manipulation                             1 2 3 4 5 6 7 8 9 1 2 3 4 5 6 7 8 9 1 2 3 4 5 6 7 8 9 1 2 3 4 5 6 7 8 9   ( 93- 96)
                                                 (5.0, 1.1, I)     (3.0, 1.4, I)     (5.0, 1.3, I)     (5.0, 2.0, I)
```

Appropriateness scale: 1 = extremely inappropriate, 5 = uncertain, 9 = extremely appropriate.

Chapter 2
CERVICAL SPINAL MANIPULATION OR MOBILIZATION IS APPROPRIATE WITH:
SUBACUTE OR CHRONIC NECK PAIN AND SIGNS OF PAINFUL AND/OR LIMITED ACTIVE RANGE OF MOTION AND PAIN ANATOMICALLY CONSISTENT WITH A MUSCULOTENDINOUS DISTRIBUTION AND
NO RADICULOPATHY AND

	NO OTHER ADEQUATE CONSERVATIVE CARE FOR THIS EPISODE		NONMANIPULATIVE CONSERVATIVE CARE FOR THIS EPISODE HAS FAILED		
	Mobilization	Manipulation	Mobilization	Manipulation	
NO CONTINUED PSYCHOSOCIAL STRESS AND					
A. Non-traumatic or minimally traumatic etiology and no prior experience with SMT AND					
1. No clinical risk factors for radiographic contraindications to cervical manipulation, and no cervical radiographs	1 6 2 1 2 3 4 5 6 7 8 9 (7.0, 0.4, A)	2 1 1 5 1 2 3 4 5 6 7 8 9 (7.0, 1.4, I)	1 5 3 1 2 3 4 5 6 7 8 9 (7.0, 0.4, A)	2 1 5 1 1 2 3 4 5 6 7 8 9 (7.0, 1.3, I)	(97-100)
2. Presence of clinical risk factors for radiographic contraindications to cervical manipulation, and no cervical radiographs	2 2 1 3 1 1 2 3 4 5 6 7 8 9 (5.0, 1.7, I)	3 1 4 1 1 2 3 4 5 6 7 8 9 (3.0, 1.0, A)	2 1 5 1 1 2 3 4 5 6 7 8 9 (6.0, 1.4, I)	2 4 1 1 1 1 2 3 4 5 6 7 8 9 (2.0, 1.1, A)	(101-104)
3. Cervical radiographs show no contraindications to cervical manipulation	4 2 3 1 2 3 4 5 6 7 8 9 (8.0, 0.8, A)	1 3 2 3 1 2 3 4 5 6 7 8 9 (8.0, 0.9, A)	3 3 3 1 2 3 4 5 6 7 8 9 (8.0, 0.7, A)	2 2 1 4 1 2 3 4 5 6 7 8 9 (8.0, 1.1, A)	(105-108)
B. Non-traumatic or minimally traumatic etiology and favorable prior experience with SMT AND					
1. No clinical risk factors for radiographic contraindications to cervical manipulation, and no cervical radiographs	1 4 2 2 1 2 3 4 5 6 7 8 9 (7.0, 0.9, A)	1 1 1 2 4 1 2 3 4 5 6 7 8 9 (6.0, 1.8, I)	2 6 1 1 2 3 4 5 6 7 8 9 (8.0, 0.3, A)	1 1 1 3 3 1 2 3 4 5 6 7 8 9 (7.0, 1.6, I)	(109-112)
2. Presence of clinical risk factors for radiographic contraindications to cervical manipulation, and no cervical radiographs	2 2 2 3 1 2 3 4 5 6 7 8 9 (5.0, 1.4, A)	2 2 3 1 1 1 2 3 4 5 6 7 8 9 (3.0, 1.0, A)	1 1 1 1 4 1 1 2 3 4 5 6 7 8 9 (6.0, 1.6, I)	2 2 2 2 1 1 2 3 4 5 6 7 8 9 (3.0, 1.2, I)	(113-116)
3. Cervical radiographs show no contraindications to cervical manipulation	4 2 3 1 2 3 4 5 6 7 8 9 (8.0, 0.8, A)	2 3 1 3 1 2 3 4 5 6 7 8 9 (7.0, 1.0, A)	2 5 2 1 2 3 4 5 6 7 8 9 (8.0, 0.4, A)	2 4 3 1 2 3 4 5 6 7 8 9 (8.0, 0.8, A)	(117-120)

Appropriateness scale: 1 = extremely inappropriate, 5 = uncertain, 9 = extremely appropriate.

- 7 - Mon Sep 25 12:29:24 1995

Chapter 2 CERVICAL SPINAL MANIPULATION OR MOBILIZATION IS APPROPRIATE WITH: SUBACUTE OR CHRONIC NECK PAIN AND SIGNS OF PAINFUL AND/OR LIMITED ACTIVE RANGE OF MOTION AND PAIN ANATOMICALLY CONSISTENT WITH A MUSCULOTENDINOUS DISTRIBUTION AND NO RADICULOPATHY AND	NO OTHER ADEQUATE CONSERVATIVE CARE FOR THIS EPISODE Mobilization	 Manipulation	NONMANIPULATIVE CONSERVATIVE CARE FOR THIS EPISODE HAS FAILED Mobilization	 Manipulation	
NO CONTINUED PSYCHOSOCIAL STRESS AND					
C. Non-traumatic or minimally traumatic etiology and no response to prior experience with SMT AND					
1. No clinical risk factors for radiographic contraindications to cervical manipulation, and no cervical radiographs	2 5 2 (at 6 7 8) 1 2 3 4 5 6 7 8 9 (7.0, 0.4, A)	1 1 4 3 (at 1 3 5 6) 1 2 3 4 5 6 7 8 9 (5.0, 1.0, A)	2 3 4 (at 5 7 8) 1 2 3 4 5 6 7 8 9 (7.0, 0.9, A)	1 1 1 3 1 2 (at 2 4 5 6 7 8) 1 2 3 4 5 6 7 8 9 (6.0, 1.3, I)	(121-124)
2. Presence of clinical risk factors for radiographic contraindications to cervical manipulation, and no cervical radiographs	1 1 2 1 2 2 (at 1 2 3 4 5 7) 1 2 3 4 5 6 7 8 9 (4.0, 1.7, I)	3 1 3 2 (at 1 2 3 5) 1 2 3 4 5 6 7 8 9 (3.0, 1.2, A)	1 1 2 1 1 2 1 (at 1 2 3 4 5 7 8) 1 2 3 4 5 6 7 8 9 (4.0, 2.0, D)	3 2 1 2 1 (at 1 2 3 5 6) 1 2 3 4 5 6 7 8 9 (2.0, 1.6, I)	(125-128)
3. Cervical radiographs show no contraindications to cervical manipulation	1 8 (at 7 8) 1 2 3 4 5 6 7 8 9 (8.0, 0.1, A)	1 3 4 1 (at 4 6 7 8) 1 2 3 4 5 6 7 8 9 (7.0, 0.8, I)	2 6 1 (at 7 8 9) 1 2 3 4 5 6 7 8 9 (8.0, 0.3, A)	3 5 1 (at 6 7 9) 1 2 3 4 5 6 7 8 9 (7.0, 0.6, I)	(129-132)
D. Non-traumatic or minimally traumatic etiology and unfavorable response to prior experience with SMT AND					
1. No clinical risk factors for radiographic contraindications to cervical manipulation, and no cervical radiographs	1 4 2 2 (at 4 5 6 7) 1 2 3 4 5 6 7 8 9 (5.0, 0.8, A)	1 2 4 2 (at 1 2 3 5) 1 2 3 4 5 6 7 8 9 (3.0, 0.9, A)	2 2 4 1 (at 3 5 6 7) 1 2 3 4 5 6 7 8 9 (6.0, 1.0, I)	1 2 1 2 1 1 1 (at 1 2 3 4 5 6 7) 1 2 3 4 5 6 7 8 9 (4.0, 1.6, I)	(133-136)
2. Presence of clinical risk factors for radiographic contraindications to cervical manipulation, and no cervical radiographs	1 3 3 1 1 (at 1 2 3 4 6) 1 2 3 4 5 6 7 8 9 (3.0, 1.0, A)	7 1 1 (at 1 2 4) 1 2 3 4 5 6 7 8 9 (1.0, 0.4, A)	1 3 3 1 1 (at 1 2 3 5 6) 1 2 3 4 5 6 7 8 9 (3.0, 1.1, A)	7 1 1 (at 1 3 5) 1 2 3 4 5 6 7 8 9 (1.0, 0.7, A)	(137-140)
3. Cervical radiographs show no contraindications to cervical manipulation	1 3 5 (at 5 6 7) 1 2 3 4 5 6 7 8 9 (7.0, 0.6, I)	5 1 2 1 (at 4 5 6 7) 1 2 3 4 5 6 7 8 9 (4.0, 0.9, A)	3 2 4 (at 5 6 7) 1 2 3 4 5 6 7 8 9 (6.0, 0.8, I)	5 3 1 (at 4 6 8) 1 2 3 4 5 6 7 8 9 (4.0, 1.1, A)	(141-144)

Appropriateness scale: 1 = extremely inappropriate, 5 = uncertain, 9 = extremely appropriate.

```
Chapter 2
CERVICAL SPINAL MANIPULATION OR MOBILIZATION
IS APPROPRIATE WITH:
SUBACUTE OR CHRONIC NECK PAIN AND SIGNS OF
PAINFUL AND/OR LIMITED ACTIVE RANGE OF MOTION    NO OTHER ADEQUATE CONSERVATIVE       NONMANIPULATIVE CONSERVATIVE CARE
AND PAIN ANATOMICALLY CONSISTENT WITH A              CARE FOR THIS EPISODE              FOR THIS EPISODE HAS FAILED
MUSCULOTENDINOUS DISTRIBUTION AND                -----------------------------------  -----------------------------------
NO RADICULOPATHY AND                             Mobilization       Manipulation       Mobilization       Manipulation

NO CONTINUED PSYCHOSOCIAL STRESS AND

E. Clinically substantial traumatic etiology
   and no prior experience with SMT AND

   1. No clinical risk factors for
      radiographic contraindications to
      cervical manipulation, and no cervical     2 1 3   1 2       3 3     3         2 1 1 1 2 1 1     4   2 1 1 1
      radiographs                                1 2 3 4 5 6 7 8 9 1 2 3 4 5 6 7 8 9 1 2 3 4 5 6 7 8 9 1 2 3 4 5 6 7 8 9     (145-148)
                                                   (3.0, 1.4, I)     (2.0, 1.3, I)     (4.0, 1.8, I)     (3.0, 1.6, I)
   2. Presence of clinical risk factors for
      radiographic contraindications to
      cervical manipulation, and no cervical     3 4 1     1       6 3               2 3 3     1       5 3 1
      radiographs                                1 2 3 4 5 6 7 8 9 1 2 3 4 5 6 7 8 9 1 2 3 4 5 6 7 8 9 1 2 3 4 5 6 7 8 9     (149-152)
                                                   (2.0, 0.9, A)     (1.0, 0.3, A)     (2.0, 1.0, A)     (1.0, 0.6, A)
   3. Cervical radiographs show no
      contraindications to cervical                  1       3 5           3 2 3 1             1 5 3           3 2 2 1 1
      manipulation                               1 2 3 4 5 6 7 8 9 1 2 3 4 5 6 7 8 9 1 2 3 4 5 6 7 8 9 1 2 3 4 5 6 7 8 9     (153-156)
                                                   (8.0, 0.9, A)     (6.0, 0.9, I)     (7.0, 0.4, A)     (6.0, 1.1, I)
F. Clinically substantial traumatic etiology
   and favorable prior experience with SMT
   AND

   1. No clinical risk factors for
      radiographic contraindications to
      cervical manipulation, and no cervical     2   2 1 1 2 1     4   1 2 2         2   2   1 3 1     4 1   2 2
      radiographs                                1 2 3 4 5 6 7 8 9 1 2 3 4 5 6 7 8 9 1 2 3 4 5 6 7 8 9 1 2 3 4 5 6 7 8 9     (157-160)
                                                   (4.0, 1.8, I)     (3.0, 1.6, I)     (5.0, 1.9, I)     (2.0, 1.6, I)
   2. Presence of clinical risk factors for
      radiographic contraindications to
      cervical manipulation, and no cervical     2 5   1   1       5 3 1             2 2 4     1       5 3 1
      radiographs                                1 2 3 4 5 6 7 8 9 1 2 3 4 5 6 7 8 9 1 2 3 4 5 6 7 8 9 1 2 3 4 5 6 7 8 9     (161-164)
                                                   (2.0, 0.9, A)     (1.0, 0.6, A)     (3.0, 1.0, A)     (1.0, 0.6, A)
   3. Cervical radiographs show no
      contraindications to cervical                      1   5 2 1       1 2 1 1 4             1   4 3 1       1 2 2   1 3
      manipulation                               1 2 3 4 5 6 7 8 9 1 2 3 4 5 6 7 8 9 1 2 3 4 5 6 7 8 9 1 2 3 4 5 6 7 8 9     (165-168)
                                                   (7.0, 0.7, A)     (7.0, 1.3, I)     (7.0, 0.8, A)     (6.0, 1.7, I)
```

Appropriateness scale: 1 = extremely inappropriate, 5 = uncertain, 9 = extremely appropriate.

Chapter 2 CERVICAL SPINAL MANIPULATION OR MOBILIZATION IS APPROPRIATE WITH: SUBACUTE OR CHRONIC NECK PAIN AND SIGNS OF PAINFUL AND/OR LIMITED ACTIVE RANGE OF MOTION AND PAIN ANATOMICALLY CONSISTENT WITH A MUSCULOTENDINOUS DISTRIBUTION AND NO RADICULOPATHY AND	NO OTHER ADEQUATE CONSERVATIVE CARE FOR THIS EPISODE		NONMANIPULATIVE CONSERVATIVE CARE FOR THIS EPISODE HAS FAILED		
	Mobilization	Manipulation	Mobilization	Manipulation	
NO CONTINUED PSYCHOSOCIAL STRESS AND					
G. Clinically substantial traumatic etiology and no response to prior experience with SMT AND					
1. No clinical risk factors for radiographic contraindications to cervical manipulation, and no cervical radiographs	2 1 3 1 1 1 1 2 3 4 5 6 7 8 9 (3.0, 1.2, I)	4 1 2 2 1 2 3 4 5 6 7 8 9 (2.0, 1.1, A)	2 2 1 2 2 1 2 3 4 5 6 7 8 9 (3.0, 1.6, I)	4 3 2 1 2 3 4 5 6 7 8 9 (3.0, 1.1, A)	(169-172)
2. Presence of clinical risk factors for radiographic contraindications to cervical manipulation, and no cervical radiographs	5 2 1 1 1 2 3 4 5 6 7 8 9 (1.0, 0.9, A)	5 4 1 2 3 4 5 6 7 8 9 (1.0, 0.4, A)	3 5 1 1 2 3 4 5 6 7 8 9 (2.0, 0.8, A)	5 4 1 2 3 4 5 6 7 8 9 (1.0, 0.4, A)	(173-176)
3. Cervical radiographs show no contraindications to cervical manipulation	1 4 3 1 1 2 3 4 5 6 7 8 9 (6.0, 0.7, I)	1 1 1 1 3 2 1 2 3 4 5 6 7 8 9 (6.0, 1.3, I)	1 1 4 3 1 2 3 4 5 6 7 8 9 (7.0, 0.7, A)	1 1 3 3 1 1 2 3 4 5 6 7 8 9 (5.0, 1.3, I)	(177-180)
H. Clinically substantial traumatic etiology and unfavorable response to prior experience with SMT AND					
1. No clinical risk factors for radiographic contraindications to cervical manipulation, and no cervical radiographs	4 3 1 1 1 2 3 4 5 6 7 8 9 (2.0, 0.8, A)	8 1 1 2 3 4 5 6 7 8 9 (1.0, 0.2, A)	3 3 1 1 1 1 2 3 4 5 6 7 8 9 (2.0, 1.0, A)	6 3 1 2 3 4 5 6 7 8 9 (1.0, 0.3, A)	(181-184)
2. Presence of clinical risk factors for radiographic contraindications to cervical manipulation, and no cervical radiographs	8 1 1 2 3 4 5 6 7 8 9 (1.0, 0.1, A)	9 1 2 3 4 5 6 7 8 9 (1.0, 0.0, A)	8 1 1 2 3 4 5 6 7 8 9 (1.0, 0.1, A)	9 1 2 3 4 5 6 7 8 9 (1.0, 0.0, A)	(185-188)
3. Cervical radiographs show no contraindications to cervical manipulation	1 4 2 2 1 2 3 4 5 6 7 8 9 (5.0, 0.9, I)	1 1 3 2 2 1 2 3 4 5 6 7 8 9 (3.0, 1.2, I)	2 4 1 2 1 2 3 4 5 6 7 8 9 (5.0, 0.8, A)	1 2 2 3 1 1 2 3 4 5 6 7 8 9 (3.0, 1.9, I)	(189-192)

Appropriateness scale: 1 = extremely inappropriate, 5 = uncertain, 9 = extremely appropriate.

Chapter 3 CERVICAL SPINAL MANIPULATION OR MOBILIZATION IS APPROPRIATE WITH: PERIPHERAL PAIN OF PROBABLE SCLEROTOGENOUS DISTRIBUTION AND	NO OTHER ADEQUATE CONSERVATIVE CARE FOR THIS EPISODE		NONMANIPULATIVE CONSERVATIVE CARE FOR THIS EPISODE HAS FAILED		
	Mobilization	Manipulation	Mobilization	Manipulation	
A. Physical findings of joint dysfunction (between C2-T1), no neurologic findings AND					

1. No clinical risk factors for radiographic contraindications to cervical manipulation, and no cervical radiographs	`        1   4 4`
	`1 2 3 4 5 6 7 8 9`
	(7.0, 0.7, A)
		`1     1 1   5 1`
		`1 2 3 4 5 6 7 8 9`
		(7.0, 1.3, I)
			`        1   3 3 2`
			`1 2 3 4 5 6 7 8 9`
			(8.0, 0.9, A)
				`1       1 3   3 1`
				`1 2 3 4 5 6 7 8 9`
				(6.0, 1.7, I)
					(1- 4)

2. Presence of clinical risk factors for radiographic contraindications to cervical manipulation, and no cervical radiographs	`1     4 1 3`
	`1 2 3 4 5 6 7 8 9`
	(4.0, 1.1, A)
		`1 1 4 1 2`
		`1 2 3 4 5 6 7 8 9`
		(3.0, 0.9, I)
			`1   1 3   2 2`
			`1 2 3 4 5 6 7 8 9`
			(4.0, 1.6, I)
				`1 3 1 2   2`
				`1 2 3 4 5 6 7 8 9`
				(3.0, 1.4, I)
					(5- 8)

3. Cervical radiographs show no contraindications to cervical manipulation	`            2 4 3`
	`1 2 3 4 5 6 7 8 9`
	(8.0, 0.6, A)
		`        1 1 1 2 4`
		`1 2 3 4 5 6 7 8 9`
		(8.0, 1.1, A)
			`            1 5 3`
			`1 2 3 4 5 6 7 8 9`
			(8.0, 0.4, A)
				`          1 2 2 4`
				`1 2 3 4 5 6 7 8 9`
				(8.0, 0.9, A)
					(9- 12)

Appropriateness scale: 1 = extremely inappropriate, 5 = uncertain, 9 = extremely appropriate.

Chapter 3 CERVICAL SPINAL MANIPULATION OR MOBILIZATION IS APPROPRIATE WITH: PERIPHERAL PAIN OF PROBABLE SCLEROTOGENOUS DISTRIBUTION AND	NO OTHER ADEQUATE CONSERVATIVE CARE FOR THIS EPISODE Mobilization	 Manipulation	NONMANIPULATIVE CONSERVATIVE CARE FOR THIS EPISODE HAS FAILED Mobilization	 Manipulation	
B. Physical findings of joint dysfunction in the upper cervical spine (occiput/C1/C2) AND					
1. No clinical risk factors for radiographic contraindications to cervical manipulation, and no cervical radiographs					
a. No neurologic symptoms or findings	1 6 2 1 2 3 4 5 6 7 8 9 (7.0, 0.4, A)	1 2 3 2 1 1 2 3 4 5 6 7 8 9 (6.0, 1.1, I)	1 1 3 4 1 2 3 4 5 6 7 8 9 (7.0, 0.8, A)	1 1 2 2 2 1 1 2 3 4 5 6 7 8 9 (7.0, 1.4, I)	(13- 16)
b. Mild post-traumatic neurologic symptoms	1 4 3 1 1 2 3 4 5 6 7 8 9 (5.0, 0.9, A)	2 2 1 1 1 2 1 2 3 4 5 6 7 8 9 (3.0, 1.9, I)	1 3 3 1 1 1 2 3 4 5 6 7 8 9 (6.0, 0.9, A)	2 1 2 1 1 2 1 2 3 4 5 6 7 8 9 (3.0, 2.0, I)	(17- 20)
2. Presence of clinical risk factors for radiographic contraindications to cervical manipulation, and no cervical radiographs					
a. No neurologic symptoms or findings	1 3 2 3 1 2 3 4 5 6 7 8 9 (4.0, 1.3, I)	3 1 3 2 1 2 3 4 5 6 7 8 9 (3.0, 1.4, A)	1 4 1 1 2 1 2 3 4 5 6 7 8 9 (3.0, 1.6, I)	2 3 2 1 1 1 2 3 4 5 6 7 8 9 (2.0, 1.2, A)	(21- 24)
b. Mild post-traumatic neurologic symptoms	2 4 2 1 1 2 3 4 5 6 7 8 9 (2.0, 1.3, I)	7 1 1 1 2 3 4 5 6 7 8 9 (1.0, 1.0, A)	1 3 2 1 1 1 1 2 3 4 5 6 7 8 9 (3.0, 1.4, I)	6 1 1 1 1 2 3 4 5 6 7 8 9 (1.0, 1.0, A)	(25- 28)
3. Cervical radiographs show no contraindications to cervical manipulation					
a. No neurologic symptoms or findings	1 5 1 2 1 2 3 4 5 6 7 8 9 (7.0, 0.8, A)	2 1 2 2 2 1 2 3 4 5 6 7 8 9 (7.0, 1.2, I)	1 1 3 2 2 1 2 3 4 5 6 7 8 9 (7.0, 1.0, A)	2 2 2 3 1 2 3 4 5 6 7 8 9 (7.0, 1.3, I)	(29- 32)
b. Mild post-traumatic neurologic symptoms	1 1 1 2 3 1 1 2 3 4 5 6 7 8 9 (6.0, 1.4, I)	3 1 1 1 1 2 1 2 3 4 5 6 7 8 9 (5.0, 2.4, D)	1 2 3 2 1 1 2 3 4 5 6 7 8 9 (6.0, 0.9, I)	2 1 1 2 1 2 1 2 3 4 5 6 7 8 9 (5.0, 2.2, D)	(33- 36)
4. Any brainstem neurologic findings	9 1 2 3 4 5 6 7 8 9 (1.0, 0.0, A)	9 1 2 3 4 5 6 7 8 9 (1.0, 0.0, A)	9 1 2 3 4 5 6 7 8 9 (1.0, 0.0, A)	9 1 2 3 4 5 6 7 8 9 (1.0, 0.0, A)	(37- 40)

Appropriateness scale: 1 = extremely inappropriate, 5 = uncertain, 9 = extremely appropriate.

Chapter 3 CERVICAL SPINAL MANIPULATION OR MOBILIZATION IS APPROPRIATE WITH: PERIPHERAL PAIN OF PROBABLE SCLEROTOGENOUS DISTRIBUTION AND	NO OTHER ADEQUATE CONSERVATIVE CARE FOR THIS EPISODE Mobilization	 Manipulation	NONMANIPULATIVE CONSERVATIVE CARE FOR THIS EPISODE HAS FAILED Mobilization	 Manipulation	
C. Physical findings of joint dysfunction in the cervical spine and pain that may indicate musculotendinous involvement of distant regions					

1. Symptoms are provoked by mechanical stress in the cervical spine and no local pathology is found	`          1 4 3 1`
	`1 2 3 4 5 6 7 8 9`
	(7.0, 0.7, A)
		`        2 2 3   2`
		`1 2 3 4 5 6 7 8 9`
		(7.0, 1.1, I)
			`            3 5 1`
			`1 2 3 4 5 6 7 8 9`
			(8.0, 0.4, A)
				`        1 2 2 2 2`
				`1 2 3 4 5 6 7 8 9`
				(7.0, 1.1, I)
					(41- 44)

2. Sypmtoms are provoked by mechanical stress in the cervical spine and local pathology is found	`1 1     2 2 2 1  `
	`1 2 3 4 5 6 7 8 9`
	(6.0, 1.7, I)
		`1 2 1   1 3   1  `
		`1 2 3 4 5 6 7 8 9`
		(5.0, 2.0, I)
			`1       1 2 4   1`
			`1 2 3 4 5 6 7 8 9`
			(7.0, 1.3, I)
				`2 1     2   3 1  `
				`1 2 3 4 5 6 7 8 9`
				(5.0, 2.2, D)
					(45- 48)

3. Symptoms are not provoked by mechanical stress in the cervical spine and local pathology is found	`2 4 2 1          `
	`1 2 3 4 5 6 7 8 9`
	(2.0, 0.7, A)
		`5 3     1        `
		`1 2 3 4 5 6 7 8 9`
		(1.0, 0.8, A)
			`2 3 1 1 2        `
			`1 2 3 4 5 6 7 8 9`
			(2.0, 1.2, I)
				`3 3 2     1      `
				`1 2 3 4 5 6 7 8 9`
				(2.0, 1.0, A)
					(49- 52)

Appropriateness scale: 1 = extremely inappropriate, 5 = uncertain, 9 = extremely appropriate.

Chapter 4 CERVICAL SPINE MANIPULATION OR MOBILIZATION IS APPROPRIATE WITH: PAIN CONSISTENT WITH MUSCULOTENDINOUS INVOLVEMENT OF THE TMJ AND	NO PRIOR SMT		FAVORABLE RESPONSE TO PRIOR SMT		NO RESPONSE TO PRIOR SMT		UNFAVORABLE RESPONSE TO PRIOR SMT		
	Mobilization	Manipulation	Mobilization	Manipulation	Mobilization	Manipulation	Mobilization	Manipulation	
A. Symptoms are provoked by mechanical stress in the cervical spine and no local pathology in the TMJ is found	3 2 3 1 1 2 3 4 5 6 7 8 9 (7.0, 1.2, I)	2 1 4 2 1 2 3 4 5 6 7 8 9 (7.0, 0.8, I)	1 2 3 3 1 2 3 4 5 6 7 8 9 (8.0, 0.8, A)	1 3 2 3 1 2 3 4 5 6 7 8 9 (8.0, 0.9, A)	1 2 1 2 2 1 1 2 3 4 5 6 7 8 9 (6.0, 1.3, I)	3 1 3 1 1 1 2 3 4 5 6 7 8 9 (6.0, 1.6, I)	2 4 2 1 1 2 3 4 5 6 7 8 9 (4.0, 1.1, A)	2 1 2 1 3 1 2 3 4 5 6 7 8 9 (3.0, 1.3, I)	(1- 8)
B. Symptoms are provoked by mechanical stress in the cervical spine and local TMJ pathology is found	1 1 2 2 3 1 2 3 4 5 6 7 8 9 (6.0, 2.0, I)	1 2 2 3 1 1 2 3 4 5 6 7 8 9 (5.0, 1.6, I)	1 1 4 2 1 1 2 3 4 5 6 7 8 9 (7.0, 1.6, A)	1 2 1 2 1 2 1 2 3 4 5 6 7 8 9 (7.0, 1.8, I)	1 1 3 1 2 1 1 2 3 4 5 6 7 8 9 (3.0, 1.7, I)	1 1 2 1 2 2 1 2 3 4 5 6 7 8 9 (4.0, 1.4, I)	2 5 2 1 2 3 4 5 6 7 8 9 (2.0, 0.7, A)	2 3 2 2 1 2 3 4 5 6 7 8 9 (2.0, 0.9, A)	(9- 16)
C. Symptoms are not provoked by mechanical stress in the cervical spine and local TMJ pathology is found	5 1 2 1 1 2 3 4 5 6 7 8 9 (1.0, 1.3, I)	6 1 2 1 2 3 4 5 6 7 8 9 (1.0, 0.8, A)	1 1 2 1 2 1 1 1 2 3 4 5 6 7 8 9 (4.0, 1.6, I)	1 3 1 2 1 1 1 2 3 4 5 6 7 8 9 (3.0, 1.8, I)	3 3 1 1 1 1 2 3 4 5 6 7 8 9 (2.0, 1.1, A)	5 1 2 1 1 2 3 4 5 6 7 8 9 (1.0, 1.2, A)	8 1 1 2 3 4 5 6 7 8 9 (1.0, 0.2, A)	8 1 1 2 3 4 5 6 7 8 9 (1.0, 0.1, A)	(17- 24)

Appropriateness scale: 1 = extremely inappropriate, 5 = uncertain, 9 = extremely appropriate.

Chapter 5
CERVICAL SPINAL MANIPULATION OR MOBILIZATION IS APPROPRIATE WITH:
ACUTE NECK PAIN AND CLINICAL SUSPICION OF CERVICAL NERVE ROOT INVOLVEMENT AND

	NO PRIOR SMT		FAVORABLE RESPONSE TO PRIOR SMT		NO RESPONSE TO PRIOR SMT		UNFAVORABLE RESPONSE TO PRIOR SMT		
	Mobilization	Manipulation	Mobilization	Manipulation	Mobilization	Manipulation	Mobilization	Manipulation	
NO CERVICAL SPINE RADIOGRAPHS									
a. Possible radiculopathy	2 5 2 1 2 3 4 5 6 7 8 9 (5.0, 0.4, A)	2 2 4 1 1 2 3 4 5 6 7 8 9 (3.0, 0.8, A)	1 5 1 2 1 2 3 4 5 6 7 8 9 (5.0, 0.7, A)	3 1 4 1 1 2 3 4 5 6 7 8 9 (4.0, 0.9, I)	2 1 4 1 1 1 2 3 4 5 6 7 8 9 (3.0, 0.9, A)	3 6 1 2 3 4 5 6 7 8 9 (2.0, 0.3, A)	5 3 1 1 2 3 4 5 6 7 8 9 (1.0, 0.6, A)	9 1 2 3 4 5 6 7 8 9 (1.0, 0.0, A)	(1- 8)
b. Definite radiculopathy	2 5 1 1 1 2 3 4 5 6 7 8 9 (2.0, 0.6, A)	8 1 1 2 3 4 5 6 7 8 9 (1.0, 0.1, A)	2 3 2 1 1 1 2 3 4 5 6 7 8 9 (2.0, 1.0, A)	6 2 1 1 2 3 4 5 6 7 8 9 (1.0, 0.4, A)	4 4 1 1 2 3 4 5 6 7 8 9 (2.0, 0.7, A)	7 2 1 2 3 4 5 6 7 8 9 (1.0, 0.2, A)	9 1 2 3 4 5 6 7 8 9 (1.0, 0.0, A)	9 1 2 3 4 5 6 7 8 9 (1.0, 0.0, A)	(9- 16)

Appropriateness scale: 1 = extremely inappropriate, 5 = uncertain, 9 = extremely appropriate.

Chapter 5 CERVICAL SPINAL MANIPULATION OR MOBILIZATION IS APPROPRIATE WITH: ACUTE NECK PAIN AND CLINICAL SUSPICION OF CERVICAL NERVE ROOT INVOLVEMENT AND	NO PRIOR SMT		FAVORABLE RESPONSE TO PRIOR SMT		NO RESPONSE TO PRIOR SMT		UNFAVORABLE RESPONSE TO PRIOR SMT		
	Mobilization	Manipulation	Mobilization	Manipulation	Mobilization	Manipulation	Mobilization	Manipulation	
NO RADIOGRAPHIC CONTRAINDICATIONS AND									
A. Non-traumatic or minimally traumatic etiology AND									
1. No advanced imaging studies AND									
a. Possible radiculopathy	1 1 3 4 1 2 3 4 5 6 7 8 9 (6.0, 0.8, I)	1 3 2 3 1 2 3 4 5 6 7 8 9 (4.0, 1.2, I)	1 8 1 2 3 4 5 6 7 8 9 (7.0, 0.1, A)	2 2 3 2 1 2 3 4 5 6 7 8 9 (6.0, 1.1, I)	1 1 1 3 3 1 2 3 4 5 6 7 8 9 (5.0, 1.2, A)	1 3 1 2 1 1 1 2 3 4 5 6 7 8 9 (3.0, 1.3, I)	1 4 1 3 1 2 3 4 5 6 7 8 9 (2.0, 0.9, I)	5 2 1 1 1 2 3 4 5 6 7 8 9 (1.0, 0.9, A)	(17- 24)
b. Definite radiculopathy	1 1 2 1 3 1 1 2 3 4 5 6 7 8 9 (5.0, 1.6, I)	4 2 1 1 1 1 2 3 4 5 6 7 8 9 (2.0, 1.3, A)	1 1 3 2 2 1 2 3 4 5 6 7 8 9 (5.0, 1.1, I)	3 2 1 1 2 1 2 3 4 5 6 7 8 9 (2.0, 1.8, I)	2 2 3 1 1 1 2 3 4 5 6 7 8 9 (4.0, 1.2, I)	5 1 1 2 1 2 3 4 5 6 7 8 9 (1.0, 1.2, A)	3 3 2 1 1 2 3 4 5 6 7 8 9 (2.0, 0.8, A)	6 1 1 1 1 2 3 4 5 6 7 8 9 (1.0, 0.7, A)	(25- 32)
2. Advanced imaging studies show no abnormalities AND									
a. Possible radiculopathy	3 6 1 2 3 4 5 6 7 8 9 (8.0, 0.3, A)	1 3 2 2 1 1 2 3 4 5 6 7 8 9 (7.0, 1.1, I)	3 5 1 1 2 3 4 5 6 7 8 9 (8.0, 0.4, A)	1 3 2 3 1 2 3 4 5 6 7 8 9 (8.0, 0.9, A)	1 5 3 1 2 3 4 5 6 7 8 9 (6.0, 0.4, I)	1 4 2 1 1 1 2 3 4 5 6 7 8 9 (5.0, 0.9, A)	2 1 6 1 2 3 4 5 6 7 8 9 (5.0, 0.6, A)	2 2 2 2 1 1 2 3 4 5 6 7 8 9 (4.0, 1.2, I)	(33- 40)
b. Definite radiculopathy	1 1 4 3 1 2 3 4 5 6 7 8 9 (6.0, 0.7, I)	1 2 3 1 2 1 2 3 4 5 6 7 8 9 (5.0, 1.3, I)	1 2 3 3 1 2 3 4 5 6 7 8 9 (7.0, 0.8, I)	1 2 3 1 1 1 1 2 3 4 5 6 7 8 9 (6.0, 1.1, I)	1 2 3 2 1 1 2 3 4 5 6 7 8 9 (5.0, 0.9, A)	1 2 1 2 2 1 1 2 3 4 5 6 7 8 9 (5.0, 1.8, I)	1 1 3 2 2 1 2 3 4 5 6 7 8 9 (3.0, 1.0, I)	2 4 1 1 1 1 2 3 4 5 6 7 8 9 (2.0, 1.2, I)	(41- 48)
3. Advanced imaging findings of cervical disc herniation AND									
a. Possible radiculopathy	1 1 4 1 2 1 2 3 4 5 6 7 8 9 (5.0, 1.0, I)	3 1 2 2 1 1 2 3 4 5 6 7 8 9 (3.0, 1.7, I)	5 1 3 1 2 3 4 5 6 7 8 9 (5.0, 0.8, I)	2 2 2 1 1 1 1 2 3 4 5 6 7 8 9 (4.0, 1.6, I)	2 3 4 1 2 3 4 5 6 7 8 9 (4.0, 1.1, A)	4 1 2 2 1 2 3 4 5 6 7 8 9 (2.0, 1.3, A)	5 2 2 1 2 3 4 5 6 7 8 9 (1.0, 1.1, A)	6 2 1 1 2 3 4 5 6 7 8 9 (1.0, 0.4, A)	(49- 56)
b. Definite radiculopathy	2 1 2 4 1 2 3 4 5 6 7 8 9 (4.0, 1.3, I)	5 1 2 1 1 2 3 4 5 6 7 8 9 (1.0, 1.4, I)	2 2 4 1 1 2 3 4 5 6 7 8 9 (5.0, 1.2, A)	4 2 1 1 1 1 2 3 4 5 6 7 8 9 (3.0, 1.6, I)	2 1 3 1 2 1 2 3 4 5 6 7 8 9 (3.0, 1.1, I)	4 3 1 1 1 2 3 4 5 6 7 8 9 (2.0, 0.8, A)	5 2 1 1 1 2 3 4 5 6 7 8 9 (1.0, 0.8, A)	8 1 1 2 3 4 5 6 7 8 9 (1.0, 0.1, A)	(57- 64)
4. Advanced imaging findings of cervical spinal canal stenosis AND									
a. Possible radiculopathy	1 4 3 1 1 2 3 4 5 6 7 8 9 (5.0, 0.8, A)	2 3 1 1 1 1 1 2 3 4 5 6 7 8 9 (2.0, 1.3, I)	1 1 2 2 1 2 1 2 3 4 5 6 7 8 9 (6.0, 1.3, I)	2 2 3 1 1 1 2 3 4 5 6 7 8 9 (3.0, 1.4, A)	1 2 3 2 1 1 2 3 4 5 6 7 8 9 (3.0, 1.3, I)	4 2 1 1 1 1 2 3 4 5 6 7 8 9 (2.0, 1.2, A)	4 3 1 1 1 2 3 4 5 6 7 8 9 (2.0, 0.8, A)	8 1 1 2 3 4 5 6 7 8 9 (1.0, 0.4, A)	(65- 72)
b. Definite radiculopathy	3 1 3 2 1 2 3 4 5 6 7 8 9 (5.0, 1.8, I)	5 1 2 1 1 2 3 4 5 6 7 8 9 (1.0, 1.0, A)	2 1 1 3 1 1 1 2 3 4 5 6 7 8 9 (5.0, 1.8, I)	5 1 1 1 1 1 2 3 4 5 6 7 8 9 (1.0, 1.4, I)	4 3 1 1 1 2 3 4 5 6 7 8 9 (2.0, 1.0, A)	5 2 1 1 1 2 3 4 5 6 7 8 9 (1.0, 0.9, A)	8 1 1 2 3 4 5 6 7 8 9 (1.0, 0.2, A)	8 1 1 2 3 4 5 6 7 8 9 (1.0, 0.3, A)	(73- 80)
5. Advanced imaging findings of cervical spinal foraminal osteophytosis AND									
a. Possible radiculopathy	2 3 4 1 2 3 4 5 6 7 8 9 (6.0, 0.7, I)	1 1 1 1 2 1 2 1 2 3 4 5 6 7 8 9 (5.0, 1.7, I)	2 2 4 1 1 2 3 4 5 6 7 8 9 (7.0, 0.8, I)	1 2 4 2 1 2 3 4 5 6 7 8 9 (6.0, 1.4, I)	1 2 2 3 1 1 2 3 4 5 6 7 8 9 (4.0, 1.1, I)	1 4 1 2 1 1 2 3 4 5 6 7 8 9 (2.0, 1.4, I)	3 3 1 1 1 1 2 3 4 5 6 7 8 9 (2.0, 1.0, A)	4 3 1 1 1 2 3 4 5 6 7 8 9 (2.0, 1.0, A)	(81- 88)
b. Definite radiculopathy	1 1 4 1 2 1 2 3 4 5 6 7 8 9 (5.0, 1.3, I)	3 2 1 1 1 1 1 2 3 4 5 6 7 8 9 (2.0, 1.9, I)	1 1 3 2 2 1 2 3 4 5 6 7 8 9 (5.0, 1.2, I)	3 1 1 1 1 1 1 1 2 3 4 5 6 7 8 9 (3.0, 1.9, I)	2 1 2 1 2 1 1 2 3 4 5 6 7 8 9 (3.0, 1.4, I)	4 2 3 1 2 3 4 5 6 7 8 9 (2.0, 1.4, I)	4 2 1 1 1 1 2 3 4 5 6 7 8 9 (2.0, 1.1, A)	6 1 2 1 2 3 4 5 6 7 8 9 (1.0, 0.8, A)	(89- 96)

Appropriateness scale: 1 = extremely inappropriate, 5 = uncertain, 9 = extremely appropriate.

Chapter 5

CERVICAL SPINAL MANIPULATION OR MOBILIZATION IS APPROPRIATE WITH: ACUTE NECK PAIN AND CLINICAL SUSPICION OF CERVICAL NERVE ROOT INVOLVEMENT AND	NO PRIOR SMT		FAVORABLE RESPONSE TO PRIOR SMT		NO RESPONSE TO PRIOR SMT		UNFAVORABLE RESPONSE TO PRIOR SMT		
	Mobilization	Manipulation	Mobilization	Manipulation	Mobilization	Manipulation	Mobilization	Manipulation	
NO RADIOGRAPHIC CONTRAINDICATIONS AND									
B. Clinically substantial traumatic etiology AND									
1. No advanced imaging studies AND									
a. Possible radiculopathy	1 1 1 4 1 1 1 2 3 4 5 6 7 8 9 (5.0, 1.1, I)	2 4 1 1 1 1 2 3 4 5 6 7 8 9 (2.0, 1.1, A)	1 1 3 3 1 1 2 3 4 5 6 7 8 9 (5.0, 1.2, I)	2 2 2 1 2 1 2 3 4 5 6 7 8 9 (3.0, 1.7, I)	1 3 2 2 1 1 2 3 4 5 6 7 8 9 (4.0, 1.1, I)	3 3 1 2 1 2 3 4 5 6 7 8 9 (2.0, 1.1, A)	4 2 1 2 1 2 3 4 5 6 7 8 9 (2.0, 1.0, A)	7 1 1 1 2 3 4 5 6 7 8 9 (1.0, 0.6, A)	(97-104)
b. Definite radiculopathy	2 1 3 2 1 1 2 3 4 5 6 7 8 9 (3.0, 1.4, I)	6 1 1 1 1 2 3 4 5 6 7 8 9 (1.0, 0.9, A)	2 2 3 2 1 2 3 4 5 6 7 8 9 (5.0, 1.6, I)	6 1 1 1 1 2 3 4 5 6 7 8 9 (1.0, 1.2, A)	3 3 2 1 1 2 3 4 5 6 7 8 9 (3.0, 1.1, I)	6 1 1 1 1 2 3 4 5 6 7 8 9 (1.0, 0.7, A)	4 2 3 1 2 3 4 5 6 7 8 9 (2.0, 0.8, A)	8 1 1 2 3 4 5 6 7 8 9 (1.0, 0.2, A)	(105-112)
2. Advanced imaging studies show no abnormalities AND									
a. Possible radiculopathy	1 5 3 1 2 3 4 5 6 7 8 9 (7.0, 0.4, A)	4 2 2 1 1 2 3 4 5 6 7 8 9 (6.0, 1.0, I)	1 3 4 1 1 2 3 4 5 6 7 8 9 (8.0, 0.7, A)	4 2 2 1 1 2 3 4 5 6 7 8 9 (7.0, 0.9, I)	2 3 3 1 1 2 3 4 5 6 7 8 9 (5.0, 0.8, A)	1 1 2 2 1 2 1 2 3 4 5 6 7 8 9 (4.0, 1.6, I)	1 3 4 1 1 2 3 4 5 6 7 8 9 (5.0, 1.6, I)	3 3 1 2 1 2 3 4 5 6 7 8 9 (2.0, 1.3, A)	(113-120)
b. Definite radiculopathy	1 1 3 3 1 1 2 3 4 5 6 7 8 9 (5.0, 1.6, I)	2 1 1 2 1 1 1 1 2 3 4 5 6 7 8 9 (5.0, 2.1, I)	2 2 1 3 1 1 2 3 4 5 6 7 8 9 (7.0, 1.9, I)	2 1 2 1 3 1 2 3 4 5 6 7 8 9 (5.0, 1.8, I)	2 1 3 3 1 2 3 4 5 6 7 8 9 (5.0, 1.4, I)	2 3 1 1 1 1 1 2 3 4 5 6 7 8 9 (2.0, 1.7, I)	5 1 3 1 2 3 4 5 6 7 8 9 (1.0, 1.7, I)	6 1 1 1 1 2 3 4 5 6 7 8 9 (1.0, 1.1, A)	(121-128)
3. Advanced imaging findings of cervical disc herniation AND									
a. Possible radiculopathy	1 1 2 3 1 1 1 2 3 4 5 6 7 8 9 (5.0, 1.3, I)	3 1 3 1 1 1 2 3 4 5 6 7 8 9 (3.0, 1.6, A)	1 1 1 4 2 1 2 3 4 5 6 7 8 9 (6.0, 1.2, I)	2 2 1 1 1 2 1 2 3 4 5 6 7 8 9 (4.0, 1.9, I)	2 3 1 2 1 1 2 3 4 5 6 7 8 9 (3.0, 1.3, I)	3 2 3 1 1 2 3 4 5 6 7 8 9 (2.0, 1.0, A)	4 3 1 1 1 2 3 4 5 6 7 8 9 (2.0, 0.9, A)	6 2 1 1 2 3 4 5 6 7 8 9 (1.0, 0.6, A)	(129-136)
b. Definite radiculopathy	2 1 1 3 2 1 2 3 4 5 6 7 8 9 (5.0, 1.4, I)	5 1 1 1 1 1 2 3 4 5 6 7 8 9 (1.0, 1.4, I)	2 1 2 3 1 1 2 3 4 5 6 7 8 9 (5.0, 1.6, I)	3 3 1 2 1 2 3 4 5 6 7 8 9 (2.0, 1.6, I)	2 2 2 3 1 2 3 4 5 6 7 8 9 (3.0, 1.0, I)	5 1 2 1 1 2 3 4 5 6 7 8 9 (1.0, 0.9, A)	5 3 1 1 2 3 4 5 6 7 8 9 (1.0, 0.6, A)	6 2 1 1 2 3 4 5 6 7 8 9 (1.0, 0.4, A)	(137-144)
4. Advanced imaging findings of cervical spinal canal stenosis AND									
a. Possible radiculopathy	1 3 1 4 1 2 3 4 5 6 7 8 9 (5.0, 1.2, A)	3 2 1 1 2 1 2 3 4 5 6 7 8 9 (2.0, 1.6, I)	1 1 2 4 1 1 2 3 4 5 6 7 8 9 (6.0, 1.1, A)	2 2 1 1 1 1 1 1 2 3 4 5 6 7 8 9 (3.0, 1.8, I)	2 3 2 2 1 2 3 4 5 6 7 8 9 (3.0, 1.1, I)	3 2 2 1 1 1 2 3 4 5 6 7 8 9 (2.0, 1.1, A)	4 1 4 1 2 3 4 5 6 7 8 9 (2.0, 0.9, A)	7 1 1 1 2 3 4 5 6 7 8 9 (1.0, 0.4, A)	(145-152)
b. Definite radiculopathy	1 2 2 3 1 1 2 3 4 5 6 7 8 9 (3.0, 1.4, I)	5 1 2 1 1 2 3 4 5 6 7 8 9 (1.0, 1.0, A)	1 1 1 4 2 1 2 3 4 5 6 7 8 9 (5.0, 1.2, I)	4 2 1 1 1 1 2 3 4 5 6 7 8 9 (2.0, 1.2, A)	3 2 2 1 1 1 2 3 4 5 6 7 8 9 (2.0, 1.1, A)	5 1 2 1 1 2 3 4 5 6 7 8 9 (1.0, 1.0, A)	6 2 1 1 2 3 4 5 6 7 8 9 (1.0, 0.4, A)	8 1 1 2 3 4 5 6 7 8 9 (1.0, 0.3, A)	(153-160)
5. Advanced imaging findings of cervical spinal foraminal osteophytosis AND									
a. Possible radiculopathy	1 3 3 2 1 2 3 4 5 6 7 8 9 (6.0, 0.9, I)	1 3 1 3 1 1 2 3 4 5 6 7 8 9 (4.0, 1.6, I)	1 1 3 3 1 1 2 3 4 5 6 7 8 9 (6.0, 1.0, I)	2 1 3 1 2 1 2 3 4 5 6 7 8 9 (5.0, 1.7, I)	1 3 3 2 1 2 3 4 5 6 7 8 9 (5.0, 1.0, A)	2 2 2 2 1 1 2 3 4 5 6 7 8 9 (3.0, 1.4, I)	1 3 1 3 1 1 2 3 4 5 6 7 8 9 (3.0, 1.1, I)	6 2 1 1 2 3 4 5 6 7 8 9 (1.0, 0.9, A)	(161-168)
b. Definite radiculopathy	2 2 2 3 1 2 3 4 5 6 7 8 9 (4.0, 1.6, I)	5 1 1 2 1 2 3 4 5 6 7 8 9 (1.0, 1.2, A)	1 2 2 3 1 1 2 3 4 5 6 7 8 9 (5.0, 1.6, I)	5 1 3 1 2 3 4 5 6 7 8 9 (1.0, 1.9, I)	3 1 1 2 2 1 2 3 4 5 6 7 8 9 (3.0, 1.4, I)	4 2 1 1 1 1 2 3 4 5 6 7 8 9 (2.0, 1.1, A)	4 1 2 2 1 2 3 4 5 6 7 8 9 (2.0, 1.1, A)	8 1 1 2 3 4 5 6 7 8 9 (1.0, 0.3, A)	(169-176)

Appropriateness scale: 1 = extremely inappropriate, 5 = uncertain, 9 = extremely appropriate.

Chapter 6 CERVICAL SPINAL MANIPULATION OR MOBILIZATION IS APPROPRIATE WITH: SUBACUTE OR CHRONIC NECK PAIN AND CLINICAL SUSPICION OF CERVICAL NERVE ROOT INVOLVEMENT AND	NO OTHER ADEQUATE CONSERVATIVE CARE FOR THIS EPISODE		NONMANIPULATIVE CONSERVATIVE CARE FOR THIS EPISODE HAS FAILED		
	Mobilization	Manipulation	Mobilization	Manipulation	
NO CERVICAL SPINE RADIOGRAPHS					
a. Possible radiculopathy	1 1 4 1 2 1 2 3 4 5 6 7 8 9 (5.0, 1.1, I)	1 3 4 1 1 2 3 4 5 6 7 8 9 (4.0, 1.1, I)	1 1 1 1 2 2 1 1 2 3 4 5 6 7 8 9 (6.0, 1.6, I)	1 3 1 1 2 1 1 2 3 4 5 6 7 8 9 (3.0, 1.4, I)	(1- 4)
b. Definite radiculopathy	3 1 4 1 1 2 3 4 5 6 7 8 9 (4.0, 1.0, I)	5 1 2 1 1 2 3 4 5 6 7 8 9 (1.0, 0.9, A)	3 1 1 3 1 1 2 3 4 5 6 7 8 9 (4.0, 1.3, I)	5 1 1 2 1 2 3 4 5 6 7 8 9 (1.0, 1.0, A)	(5- 8)

Appropriateness scale: 1 = extremely inappropriate, 5 = uncertain, 9 = extremely appropriate.

```
Chapter 6
CERVICAL SPINAL MANIPULATION OR MOBILIZATION
IS APPROPRIATE WITH:                    NO OTHER ADEQUATE CONSERVATIVE          NONMANIPULATIVE CONSERVATIVE CARE
SUBACUTE OR CHRONIC NECK PAIN AND CLINICAL   CARE FOR THIS EPISODE               FOR THIS EPISODE HAS FAILED
SUSPICION OF CERVICAL NERVE ROOT INVOLVEMENT ---------------------------------   ---------------------------------
AND                                     Mobilization         Manipulation        Mobilization         Manipulation

NO RADIOGRAPHIC CONTRAINDICATIONS AND

A. Non-traumatic or minimally traumatic
   etiology and no prior history of SMT AND

   1. No advanced imaging studies AND
                                                2 2 5         2 1 2 1 1 2            2 2 3 2     2     4   2 1
      a. Possible Radiculopathy         1 2 3 4 5 6 7 8 9   1 2 3 4 5 6 7 8 9   1 2 3 4 5 6 7 8 9   1 2 3 4 5 6 7 8 9     ( 9- 12)
                                         (7.0, 0.7, I)       (4.0, 1.6, I)       (7.0, 0.9, I)       (5.0, 1.4, I)

                                        1 1   1 3 3         4   2   2   1       1   2   2 3   1     2 1 2   1 2 1
      b. Definite radiculopathy         1 2 3 4 5 6 7 8 9   1 2 3 4 5 6 7 8 9   1 2 3 4 5 6 7 8 9   1 2 3 4 5 6 7 8 9     ( 13- 16)
                                         (5.0, 1.2, A)       (3.0, 1.8, I)       (5.0, 1.6, I)       (3.0, 1.9, I)
   2. Advanced imaging studies show no
      abnormalities AND
                                                  1 2 6             3 1 2 3               1 2 5 1           1 3 2   3
      a. Possible Radiculopathy         1 2 3 4 5 6 7 8 9   1 2 3 4 5 6 7 8 9   1 2 3 4 5 6 7 8 9   1 2 3 4 5 6 7 8 9     ( 17- 20)
                                         (8.0, 0.4, A)       (7.0, 1.1, I)       (8.0, 0.6, A)       (7.0, 1.2, I)

                                            2     2 3 2     1   2   2 1 3           1 1 2     5     1   2 1 1 1 2 1
      b. Definite radiculopathy         1 2 3 4 5 6 7 8 9   1 2 3 4 5 6 7 8 9   1 2 3 4 5 6 7 8 9   1 2 3 4 5 6 7 8 9     ( 21- 24)
                                         (7.0, 1.3, I)       (5.0, 1.7, D)       (8.0, 1.7, I)       (5.0, 1.9, D)
   3. Advanced imaging findings of cervical
      disc herniation AND
                                            1 1 4 3         4   1 1   2 1           1 1 3 1 3       3 1 1 1     3
      a. Possible Radiculopathy         1 2 3 4 5 6 7 8 9   1 2 3 4 5 6 7 8 9   1 2 3 4 5 6 7 8 9   1 2 3 4 5 6 7 8 9     ( 25- 28)
                                         (5.0, 0.7, A)       (3.0, 2.1, I)       (5.0, 1.1, I)       (3.0, 2.2, D)

                                        2   1 2 3 1         4 2     2 1         2   1   3 1 2       4 2       3
      b. Definite radiculopathy         1 2 3 4 5 6 7 8 9   1 2 3 4 5 6 7 8 9   1 2 3 4 5 6 7 8 9   1 2 3 4 5 6 7 8 9     ( 29- 32)
                                         (4.0, 1.3, I)       (2.0, 1.6, I)       (5.0, 1.7, I)       (2.0, 1.8, I)
   4. Advanced imaging findings of cervical
      spinal canal stenosis AND
                                        1     3 2 2 1       2 3   1 2   1       1     4   2 2       2 3   1   2   1
      a. Possible Radiculopathy         1 2 3 4 5 6 7 8 9   1 2 3 4 5 6 7 8 9   1 2 3 4 5 6 7 8 9   1 2 3 4 5 6 7 8 9     ( 33- 36)
                                         (5.0, 1.2, A)       (2.0, 1.7, I)       (4.0, 1.4, I)       (2.0, 2.0, I)

                                        2   2 1 3 1         4 2   1 1 1         2 1 1 1 1 2 1       4 2   1   1 1
      b. Definite radiculopathy         1 2 3 4 5 6 7 8 9   1 2 3 4 5 6 7 8 9   1 2 3 4 5 6 7 8 9   1 2 3 4 5 6 7 8 9     ( 37- 40)
                                         (4.0, 1.4, I)       (2.0, 1.4, I)       (4.0, 1.9, I)       (2.0, 1.7, I)
   5. Advanced imaging findings of cervical
      spinal foraminal osteophytosis AND
                                              2 2 4 1       2 1 1 1 1 1 2             2 3   4       1 1 2 1 1 1 1 1
      a. Possible Radiculopathy         1 2 3 4 5 6 7 8 9   1 2 3 4 5 6 7 8 9   1 2 3 4 5 6 7 8 9   1 2 3 4 5 6 7 8 9     ( 41- 44)
                                         (6.0, 0.8, A)       (4.0, 2.0, I)       (5.0, 1.1, I)       (4.0, 1.9, I)

                                        2   1 2 3 1         4 1 1 1   2         2   2   1 2 2       4 2     1   2
      b. Definite radiculopathy         1 2 3 4 5 6 7 8 9   1 2 3 4 5 6 7 8 9   1 2 3 4 5 6 7 8 9   1 2 3 4 5 6 7 8 9     ( 45- 48)
                                         (4.0, 1.3, I)       (2.0, 1.7, I)       (5.0, 2.0, I)       (2.0, 1.9, I)
```

Appropriateness scale: 1 = extremely inappropriate, 5 = uncertain, 9 = extremely appropriate.

Chapter 6

CERVICAL SPINAL MANIPULATION OR MOBILIZATION IS APPROPRIATE WITH: SUBACUTE OR CHRONIC NECK PAIN AND CLINICAL SUSPICION OF CERVICAL NERVE ROOT INVOLVEMENT AND	NO OTHER ADEQUATE CONSERVATIVE CARE FOR THIS EPISODE		NONMANIPULATIVE CONSERVATIVE CARE FOR THIS EPISODE HAS FAILED		
	Mobilization	Manipulation	Mobilization	Manipulation	
NO RADIOGRAPHIC CONTRAINDICATIONS AND					
B. Non-traumatic or minimally traumatic etiology and favorable prior experience with SMT AND					
1. No advanced imaging studies AND					
a. Possible Radiculopathy	1 3 4 1 1 2 3 4 5 6 7 8 9 (7.0, 0.7, I)	2 1 3 2 1 1 2 3 4 5 6 7 8 9 (5.0, 1.3, I)	2 2 2 3 1 2 3 4 5 6 7 8 9 (7.0, 1.0, I)	1 1 3 1 3 1 2 3 4 5 6 7 8 9 (5.0, 1.7, I)	(49- 52)
b. Definite radiculopathy	1 1 1 2 3 1 1 2 3 4 5 6 7 8 9 (5.0, 1.2, I)	2 2 2 1 2 1 2 3 4 5 6 7 8 9 (3.0, 1.6, I)	2 1 2 1 1 2 1 2 3 4 5 6 7 8 9 (5.0, 1.6, I)	2 2 1 1 1 1 1 1 2 3 4 5 6 7 8 9 (3.0, 2.1, I)	(53- 56)
2. Advanced imaging studies show no abnormalities AND					
a. Possible Radiculopathy	1 2 6 1 2 3 4 5 6 7 8 9 (8.0, 0.4, A)	1 3 2 2 1 1 2 3 4 5 6 7 8 9 (7.0, 1.0, I)	1 2 4 2 1 2 3 4 5 6 7 8 9 (8.0, 0.7, A)	2 2 2 3 1 2 3 4 5 6 7 8 9 (7.0, 1.3, I)	(57- 60)
b. Definite radiculopathy	4 2 3 1 2 3 4 5 6 7 8 9 (7.0, 1.2, I)	1 1 1 2 2 2 1 2 3 4 5 6 7 8 9 (5.0, 1.6, I)	3 1 1 4 1 2 3 4 5 6 7 8 9 (7.0, 1.2, I)	1 2 1 1 1 1 2 1 2 3 4 5 6 7 8 9 (5.0, 1.9, D)	(61- 64)
3. Advanced imaging findings of cervical disc herniation AND					
a. Possible Radiculopathy	1 1 2 3 2 1 2 3 4 5 6 7 8 9 (6.0, 1.1, I)	3 1 1 1 1 1 1 1 2 3 4 5 6 7 8 9 (3.0, 2.3, I)	1 4 1 2 1 1 2 3 4 5 6 7 8 9 (5.0, 1.2, I)	1 3 1 1 1 2 1 2 3 4 5 6 7 8 9 (3.0, 2.1, I)	(65- 68)
b. Definite radiculopathy	2 2 3 2 1 2 3 4 5 6 7 8 9 (5.0, 1.3, A)	4 1 1 1 1 1 1 2 3 4 5 6 7 8 9 (2.0, 1.9, I)	2 1 2 2 1 1 1 2 3 4 5 6 7 8 9 (4.0, 2.0, I)	3 3 1 1 1 1 2 3 4 5 6 7 8 9 (2.0, 2.0, I)	(69- 72)
4. Advanced imaging findings of cervical spinal canal stenosis AND					
a. Possible Radiculopathy	1 2 1 2 3 1 2 3 4 5 6 7 8 9 (5.0, 1.3, I)	2 2 1 1 1 1 1 1 2 3 4 5 6 7 8 9 (3.0, 1.9, I)	1 1 1 2 1 3 1 2 3 4 5 6 7 8 9 (5.0, 1.6, I)	2 2 1 1 1 1 1 1 2 3 4 5 6 7 8 9 (3.0, 2.1, I)	(73- 76)
b. Definite radiculopathy	2 1 2 1 3 1 2 3 4 5 6 7 8 9 (3.0, 1.3, I)	5 1 2 1 1 2 3 4 5 6 7 8 9 (1.0, 1.7, I)	2 1 1 1 4 1 2 3 4 5 6 7 8 9 (5.0, 1.9, I)	5 1 1 1 1 1 2 3 4 5 6 7 8 9 (1.0, 1.8, I)	(77- 80)
5. Advanced imaging findings of cervical spinal foraminal osteophytosis AND					
a. Possible Radiculopathy	1 1 2 3 2 1 2 3 4 5 6 7 8 9 (6.0, 1.0, I)	1 2 1 1 1 1 1 1 1 2 3 4 5 6 7 8 9 (4.0, 2.0, I)	1 2 2 4 1 2 3 4 5 6 7 8 9 (6.0, 0.9, I)	4 2 2 1 1 2 3 4 5 6 7 8 9 (5.0, 2.1, D)	(81- 84)
b. Definite radiculopathy	1 1 1 1 2 3 1 2 3 4 5 6 7 8 9 (5.0, 1.4, I)	4 1 1 2 1 1 2 3 4 5 6 7 8 9 (2.0, 2.1, I)	1 2 1 1 3 1 1 2 3 4 5 6 7 8 9 (5.0, 1.8, I)	5 1 1 2 1 2 3 4 5 6 7 8 9 (1.0, 2.1, I)	(85- 88)

Appropriateness scale: 1 = extremely inappropriate, 5 = uncertain, 9 = extremely appropriate.

Chapter 6 CERVICAL SPINAL MANIPULATION OR MOBILIZATION IS APPROPRIATE WITH: SUBACUTE OR CHRONIC NECK PAIN AND CLINICAL SUSPICION OF CERVICAL NERVE ROOT INVOLVEMENT AND	NO OTHER ADEQUATE CONSERVATIVE CARE FOR THIS EPISODE Mobilization	 Manipulation	NONMANIPULATIVE CONSERVATIVE CARE FOR THIS EPISODE HAS FAILED Mobilization	 Manipulation	
NO RADIOGRAPHIC CONTRAINDICATIONS AND					
C. Non-traumatic or minimally traumatic etiology and no response to prior SMT AND					
1. No advanced imaging studies AND					
a. Possible Radiculopathy	1 1 1 3 1 2 1 2 3 4 5 6 7 8 9 (5.0, 1.2, I)	2 1 1 2 1 1 1 1 2 3 4 5 6 7 8 9 (4.0, 1.7, I)	1 2 2 1 2 1 1 2 3 4 5 6 7 8 9 (5.0, 1.4, I)	2 1 2 2 2 1 2 3 4 5 6 7 8 9 (3.0, 2.1, I)	(89- 92)
b. Definite radiculopathy	1 3 2 1 2 1 2 3 4 5 6 7 8 9 (4.0, 1.2, I)	2 4 1 2 1 2 3 4 5 6 7 8 9 (2.0, 1.0, A)	1 1 2 3 2 1 2 3 4 5 6 7 8 9 (5.0, 1.3, I)	2 4 3 1 2 3 4 5 6 7 8 9 (2.0, 1.6, I)	(93- 96)
2. Advanced imaging studies show no abnormalities AND					
a. Possible Radiculopathy	1 2 2 4 1 2 3 4 5 6 7 8 9 (6.0, 1.4, I)	1 2 2 1 1 2 1 2 3 4 5 6 7 8 9 (5.0, 1.8, D)	3 1 1 4 1 2 3 4 5 6 7 8 9 (7.0, 1.2, I)	1 2 1 1 1 2 1 1 2 3 4 5 6 7 8 9 (5.0, 2.1, D)	(97-100)
b. Definite radiculopathy	1 2 3 1 2 1 2 3 4 5 6 7 8 9 (5.0, 1.2, I)	1 1 3 1 1 2 1 2 3 4 5 6 7 8 9 (3.0, 1.8, I)	2 1 2 1 1 2 1 2 3 4 5 6 7 8 9 (5.0, 1.6, I)	2 1 2 1 1 2 1 2 3 4 5 6 7 8 9 (3.0, 2.3, D)	(101-104)
3. Advanced imaging findings of cervical disc herniation AND					
a. Possible Radiculopathy	1 1 2 2 2 1 1 2 3 4 5 6 7 8 9 (4.0, 1.2, I)	2 3 2 2 1 2 3 4 5 6 7 8 9 (2.0, 1.3, A)	1 1 1 2 1 2 1 1 2 3 4 5 6 7 8 9 (4.0, 1.6, I)	2 3 1 1 2 1 2 3 4 5 6 7 8 9 (2.0, 1.9, I)	(105-108)
b. Definite radiculopathy	2 2 2 1 2 1 2 3 4 5 6 7 8 9 (3.0, 1.2, I)	4 3 2 1 2 3 4 5 6 7 8 9 (2.0, 1.1, A)	2 1 2 3 1 1 2 3 4 5 6 7 8 9 (3.0, 1.7, I)	5 1 1 2 1 2 3 4 5 6 7 8 9 (1.0, 1.7, I)	(109-112)
4. Advanced imaging findings of cervical spinal canal stenosis AND					
a. Possible Radiculopathy	1 1 4 3 1 2 3 4 5 6 7 8 9 (3.0, 1.0, I)	2 4 2 1 1 2 3 4 5 6 7 8 9 (2.0, 1.3, I)	1 2 2 1 2 1 1 2 3 4 5 6 7 8 9 (3.0, 1.7, I)	2 4 1 1 1 1 2 3 4 5 6 7 8 9 (2.0, 1.7, I)	(113-116)
b. Definite radiculopathy	2 4 1 2 1 2 3 4 5 6 7 8 9 (2.0, 1.1, I)	6 2 1 1 2 3 4 5 6 7 8 9 (1.0, 1.1, I)	2 3 1 1 2 1 2 3 4 5 6 7 8 9 (2.0, 1.6, I)	6 2 1 1 2 3 4 5 6 7 8 9 (1.0, 1.3, I)	(117-120)
5. Advanced imaging findings of cervical spinal foraminal osteophytosis AND					
a. Possible Radiculopathy	2 1 5 1 1 2 3 4 5 6 7 8 9 (5.0, 0.8, I)	2 2 1 2 1 1 1 2 3 4 5 6 7 8 9 (3.0, 1.7, I)	3 3 3 1 2 3 4 5 6 7 8 9 (5.0, 1.0, I)	1 3 1 1 1 1 1 1 2 3 4 5 6 7 8 9 (4.0, 2.1, I)	(121-124)
b. Definite radiculopathy	2 2 1 3 1 1 2 3 4 5 6 7 8 9 (3.0, 1.3, I)	5 2 1 1 1 2 3 4 5 6 7 8 9 (1.0, 1.4, A)	2 1 2 1 1 2 1 2 3 4 5 6 7 8 9 (3.0, 1.9, I)	5 1 1 2 1 2 3 4 5 6 7 8 9 (1.0, 2.0, I)	(125-128)

Appropriateness scale: 1 = extremely inappropriate, 5 = uncertain, 9 = extremely appropriate.

Chapter 6 CERVICAL SPINAL MANIPULATION OR MOBILIZATION IS APPROPRIATE WITH: SUBACUTE OR CHRONIC NECK PAIN AND CLINICAL SUSPICION OF CERVICAL NERVE ROOT INVOLVEMENT AND	NO OTHER ADEQUATE CONSERVATIVE CARE FOR THIS EPISODE		NONMANIPULATIVE CONSERVATIVE CARE FOR THIS EPISODE HAS FAILED		
	Mobilization	Manipulation	Mobilization	Manipulation	
D. Non-traumatic or minimally traumatic etiology and unfavorable response to prior SMT AND					
1. No advanced imaging studies AND					
a. Possible Radiculopathy	4 1 3 1 1 2 3 4 5 6 7 8 9 (4.0, 1.4, I)	4 2 1 2 1 2 3 4 5 6 7 8 9 (2.0, 1.2, A)	2 2 2 3 1 2 3 4 5 6 7 8 9 (5.0, 1.4, I)	5 2 1 1 1 2 3 4 5 6 7 8 9 (1.0, 1.7, I)	(129-132)
b. Definite radiculopathy	3 2 1 3 1 2 3 4 5 6 7 8 9 (2.0, 1.4, I)	6 1 1 1 1 2 3 4 5 6 7 8 9 (1.0, 0.7, A)	2 1 2 1 1 2 1 2 3 4 5 6 7 8 9 (3.0, 1.6, I)	6 1 1 1 1 2 3 4 5 6 7 8 9 (1.0, 0.9, A)	(133-136)
2. Advanced imaging studies show no abnormalities AND					
a. Possible Radiculopathy	3 1 3 2 1 2 3 4 5 6 7 8 9 (5.0, 1.2, I)	1 2 2 1 1 1 1 1 2 3 4 5 6 7 8 9 (3.0, 1.6, I)	2 4 1 2 1 2 3 4 5 6 7 8 9 (5.0, 1.0, I)	1 3 1 1 2 1 1 2 3 4 5 6 7 8 9 (3.0, 1.9, I)	(137-140)
b. Definite radiculopathy	1 2 1 2 2 1 1 2 3 4 5 6 7 8 9 (4.0, 1.3, I)	4 1 1 1 1 1 1 2 3 4 5 6 7 8 9 (2.0, 1.6, I)	1 2 1 1 2 1 1 1 2 3 4 5 6 7 8 9 (4.0, 1.7, I)	5 1 1 1 1 1 2 3 4 5 6 7 8 9 (1.0, 1.8, I)	(141-144)
3. Advanced imaging findings of cervical disc herniation AND					
a. Possible Radiculopathy	4 2 2 1 1 2 3 4 5 6 7 8 9 (2.0, 1.0, A)	7 1 1 1 2 3 4 5 6 7 8 9 (1.0, 0.8, A)	3 2 1 1 1 1 1 2 3 4 5 6 7 8 9 (2.0, 1.4, I)	6 1 1 1 1 2 3 4 5 6 7 8 9 (1.0, 1.2, A)	(145-148)
b. Definite radiculopathy	6 2 1 1 2 3 4 5 6 7 8 9 (1.0, 0.6, A)	7 1 1 1 2 3 4 5 6 7 8 9 (1.0, 0.6, A)	5 1 2 1 1 2 3 4 5 6 7 8 9 (1.0, 1.3, I)	6 1 1 1 1 2 3 4 5 6 7 8 9 (1.0, 0.9, A)	(149-152)
4. Advanced imaging findings of cervical spinal canal stenosis AND					
a. Possible Radiculopathy	5 1 3 1 2 3 4 5 6 7 8 9 (1.0, 1.1, I)	6 1 1 1 1 2 3 4 5 6 7 8 9 (1.0, 0.8, A)	5 1 1 1 1 1 2 3 4 5 6 7 8 9 (1.0, 1.3, A)	7 1 1 1 2 3 4 5 6 7 8 9 (1.0, 1.0, A)	(153-156)
b. Definite radiculopathy	6 1 2 1 2 3 4 5 6 7 8 9 (1.0, 0.9, A)	7 1 1 1 2 3 4 5 6 7 8 9 (1.0, 0.4, A)	6 1 1 1 1 2 3 4 5 6 7 8 9 (1.0, 0.9, A)	7 1 1 1 2 3 4 5 6 7 8 9 (1.0, 0.7, A)	(157-160)
5. Advanced imaging findings of cervical spinal foraminal osteophytosis AND					
a. Possible Radiculopathy	1 1 4 2 1 1 2 3 4 5 6 7 8 9 (3.0, 0.9, I)	4 3 2 1 2 3 4 5 6 7 8 9 (2.0, 1.1, A)	1 2 3 3 1 2 3 4 5 6 7 8 9 (3.0, 1.4, I)	4 1 2 1 1 1 2 3 4 5 6 7 8 9 (2.0, 1.6, A)	(161-164)
b. Definite radiculopathy	5 1 2 1 1 2 3 4 5 6 7 8 9 (1.0, 1.0, A)	6 1 2 1 2 3 4 5 6 7 8 9 (1.0, 0.8, A)	4 2 1 2 1 2 3 4 5 6 7 8 9 (2.0, 1.7, I)	6 1 1 1 1 2 3 4 5 6 7 8 9 (1.0, 1.2, A)	(165-168)

Appropriateness scale: 1 = extremely inappropriate, 5 = uncertain, 9 = extremely appropriate.

```
Chapter 6
CERVICAL SPINAL MANIPULATION OR MOBILIZATION
IS APPROPRIATE WITH:                            NO OTHER ADEQUATE CONSERVATIVE        NONMANIPULATIVE CONSERVATIVE CARE
SUBACUTE OR CHRONIC NECK PAIN AND CLINICAL           CARE FOR THIS EPISODE             FOR THIS EPISODE HAS FAILED
SUSPICION OF CERVICAL NERVE ROOT INVOLVEMENT    -----------------------------------  -----------------------------------
AND                                               Mobilization       Manipulation      Mobilization       Manipulation
---------------------------------------------------------------------------------------------------------------------------
NO RADIOGRAPHIC CONTRAINDICATIONS AND

E. Clinically substantial traumatic etiology
   and no prior SMT AND

   1. No advanced imaging studies AND
                                                  2   2 3 1 1      3 1 2   1   2        2 1   2 3 1      3 1 2   1   2
      a. Possible Radiculopathy                 1 2 3 4 5 6 7 8 9  1 2 3 4 5 6 7 8 9  1 2 3 4 5 6 7 8 9  1 2 3 4 5 6 7 8 9      (169-172)
                                                  (5.0, 1.2, I)      (3.0, 1.9, I)      (5.0, 1.4, I)      (3.0, 1.9, I)

                                                2 1   3 2   1      4 2     1 1 1      2 1     5   1      4 2 1     1 1
      b. Definite radiculopathy                 1 2 3 4 5 6 7 8 9  1 2 3 4 5 6 7 8 9  1 2 3 4 5 6 7 8 9  1 2 3 4 5 6 7 8 9      (173-176)
                                                  (4.0, 1.4, I)      (2.0, 1.4, I)      (5.0, 1.4, I)      (2.0, 1.6, A)
   2. Advanced imaging studies show no
      abnormalities AND
                                                    1 2     4 2      1 2   1 2 1 1 1            3 1 1 4          2   4   1   2
      a. Possible Radiculopathy                 1 2 3 4 5 6 7 8 9  1 2 3 4 5 6 7 8 9  1 2 3 4 5 6 7 8 9  1 2 3 4 5 6 7 8 9      (177-180)
                                                  (7.0, 1.3, I)      (6.0, 1.9, D)      (7.0, 1.2, I)      (5.0, 1.6, I)

                                                1 1 1     2 2 2    2 1   1 2 1 1 1        2 2   1   4    1 1 2 1 1 1 1 1
      b. Definite radiculopathy                 1 2 3 4 5 6 7 8 9  1 2 3 4 5 6 7 8 9  1 2 3 4 5 6 7 8 9  1 2 3 4 5 6 7 8 9      (181-184)
                                                  (6.0, 2.0, D)      (5.0, 2.0, I)      (6.0, 2.0, I)      (4.0, 1.9, I)
   3. Advanced imaging findings of cervical
      disc herniation AND
                                                1   2 1 3 2        2 3 1   1 1 1      1   1 2   4 1      3 2 1     1 1 1
      a. Possible Radiculopathy                 1 2 3 4 5 6 7 8 9  1 2 3 4 5 6 7 8 9  1 2 3 4 5 6 7 8 9  1 2 3 4 5 6 7 8 9      (185-188)
                                                  (5.0, 1.2, I)      (2.0, 1.7, I)      (6.0, 1.4, I)      (2.0, 2.1, I)

                                                2 1 2 1 3          5 1   1 1 1        2 2   1 1 2 1      6     1   1 1
      b. Definite radiculopathy                 1 2 3 4 5 6 7 8 9  1 2 3 4 5 6 7 8 9  1 2 3 4 5 6 7 8 9  1 2 3 4 5 6 7 8 9      (189-192)
                                                  (3.0, 1.3, I)      (1.0, 1.4, I)      (4.0, 2.0, I)      (1.0, 1.6, I)
   4. Advanced imaging findings of cervical
      spinal canal stenosis AND
                                                1 1 1 2 1 3        4 1 1   2   1      1 1 1 1 1 3 1      4 2       2   1
      a. Possible Radiculopathy                 1 2 3 4 5 6 7 8 9  1 2 3 4 5 6 7 8 9  1 2 3 4 5 6 7 8 9  1 2 3 4 5 6 7 8 9      (193-196)
                                                  (4.0, 1.4, I)      (2.0, 1.8, I)      (5.0, 1.7, I)      (2.0, 2.0, I)

                                                2 2   2 3          6   1 1   1        3 1   2 2 1        6   1 1     1
      b. Definite radiculopathy                 1 2 3 4 5 6 7 8 9  1 2 3 4 5 6 7 8 9  1 2 3 4 5 6 7 8 9  1 2 3 4 5 6 7 8 9      (197-200)
                                                  (4.0, 1.4, I)      (1.0, 1.1, A)      (4.0, 1.7, I)      (1.0, 1.2, A)
   5. Advanced imaging findings of cervical
      spinal foraminal osteophytosis AND
                                                  1 2   2 4        4 1   1 1 1 1      1 1   2 1 1 3      4 1 1         2 1
      a. Possible Radiculopathy                 1 2 3 4 5 6 7 8 9  1 2 3 4 5 6 7 8 9  1 2 3 4 5 6 7 8 9  1 2 3 4 5 6 7 8 9      (201-204)
                                                  (5.0, 1.2, I)      (2.0, 2.0, I)      (5.0, 1.8, I)      (2.0, 2.3, D)

                                                3   1   4 1        5 1   1   2        3 1     2 2 1      6             1 2
      b. Definite radiculopathy                 1 2 3 4 5 6 7 8 9  1 2 3 4 5 6 7 8 9  1 2 3 4 5 6 7 8 9  1 2 3 4 5 6 7 8 9      (205-208)
                                                  (5.0, 1.7, I)      (1.0, 1.6, I)      (5.0, 2.1, I)      (1.0, 1.9, I)
```

Appropriateness scale: 1 = extremely inappropriate, 5 = uncertain, 9 = extremely appropriate.

```
Chapter 6
CERVICAL SPINAL MANIPULATION OR MOBILIZATION
IS APPROPRIATE WITH:                      NO OTHER ADEQUATE CONSERVATIVE         NONMANIPULATIVE CONSERVATIVE CARE
SUBACUTE OR CHRONIC NECK PAIN AND CLINICAL      CARE FOR THIS EPISODE              FOR THIS EPISODE HAS FAILED
SUSPICION OF CERVICAL NERVE ROOT INVOLVEMENT  ------------------------------------  ------------------------------------
AND                                     Mobilization       Manipulation       Mobilization       Manipulation

NO RADIOGRAPHIC CONTRAINDICATIONS AND

F. Clinically substantial traumatic etiology
   and favorable prior experience with SMT
   AND

  1. No advanced imaging studies AND
                                        1 1     4 1 2      3   2 1 1   2      1 1   1 2 2 2      3 1 1 1   1 2
    a. Possible Radiculopathy           1 2 3 4 5 6 7 8 9  1 2 3 4 5 6 7 8 9  1 2 3 4 5 6 7 8 9  1 2 3 4 5 6 7 8 9   (209-212)
                                          (5.0, 1.3, I)      (3.0, 1.9, I)      (5.0, 1.6, I)      (3.0, 2.1, I)

                                        1 1   3 2 1 1      4   2 1   2        1 1 1   4 1 1      4 1 1 1   1 1
    b. Definite radiculopathy           1 2 3 4 5 6 7 8 9  1 2 3 4 5 6 7 8 9  1 2 3 4 5 6 7 8 9  1 2 3 4 5 6 7 8 9   (213-216)
                                          (4.0, 1.3, I)      (3.0, 1.7, I)      (5.0, 1.3, I)      (2.0, 1.8, I)
  2. Advanced imaging studies show no
     abnormalities AND
                                            2     2 3 2    1   1 1 3   1 1 1          3 1   4 1          2 2 2 1   2
    a. Possible Radiculopathy           1 2 3 4 5 6 7 8 9  1 2 3 4 5 6 7 8 9  1 2 3 4 5 6 7 8 9  1 2 3 4 5 6 7 8 9   (217-220)
                                          (7.0, 1.3, I)      (5.0, 1.8, I)      (8.0, 1.3, I)      (6.0, 1.4, I)

                                        1 1   2   1 2 2    2   3   1 1 1 1    1   2   1   1 3 1  2 1 1   2 1 1 1
    b. Definite radiculopathy           1 2 3 4 5 6 7 8 9  1 2 3 4 5 6 7 8 9  1 2 3 4 5 6 7 8 9  1 2 3 4 5 6 7 8 9   (221-224)
                                          (6.0, 2.1, I)      (3.0, 2.0, I)      (7.0, 2.3, D)      (5.0, 2.1, I)
  3. Advanced imaging findings of cervical
     disc herniation AND
                                        1   1 2 2 3        2 2 1 1 1 1 1      1   1 1 2 2 2      2 3 1     1 1 1
    a. Possible Radiculopathy           1 2 3 4 5 6 7 8 9  1 2 3 4 5 6 7 8 9  1 2 3 4 5 6 7 8 9  1 2 3 4 5 6 7 8 9   (225-228)
                                          (5.0, 1.2, A)      (3.0, 1.8, I)      (5.0, 1.4, I)      (2.0, 2.0, I)

                                        2 1 1 1 4          4 2   1 1 1        2 1   1 2 2 1      5 1   1     2
    b. Definite radiculopathy           1 2 3 4 5 6 7 8 9  1 2 3 4 5 6 7 8 9  1 2 3 4 5 6 7 8 9  1 2 3 4 5 6 7 8 9   (229-232)
                                          (4.0, 1.4, I)      (2.0, 1.4, I)      (5.0, 1.8, I)      (1.0, 1.8, I)
  4. Advanced imaging findings of cervical
     spinal canal stenosis AND
                                        1   1 3 1 3        2 3 1   2     1    1   1 1 2 2 2      3 3       2     1
    a. Possible Radiculopathy           1 2 3 4 5 6 7 8 9  1 2 3 4 5 6 7 8 9  1 2 3 4 5 6 7 8 9  1 2 3 4 5 6 7 8 9   (233-236)
                                          (4.0, 1.2, A)      (2.0, 1.7, I)      (5.0, 1.4, I)      (2.0, 2.0, I)

                                        1 1 2 1 4          6     1 1   1      2 1 1   2 2 1      6       1 1     1
    b. Definite radiculopathy           1 2 3 4 5 6 7 8 9  1 2 3 4 5 6 7 8 9  1 2 3 4 5 6 7 8 9  1 2 3 4 5 6 7 8 9   (237-240)
                                          (4.0, 1.2, I)      (1.0, 1.4, I)      (5.0, 1.9, I)      (1.0, 1.6, I)
  5. Advanced imaging findings of cervical
     spinal foraminal osteophytosis AND
                                            2 1 2 3 1      2 3   1 1 1   1          3 2   4      1 4 1       2   1
    a. Possible Radiculopathy           1 2 3 4 5 6 7 8 9  1 2 3 4 5 6 7 8 9  1 2 3 4 5 6 7 8 9  1 2 3 4 5 6 7 8 9   (241-244)
                                          (5.0, 1.1, I)      (2.0, 1.9, I)      (5.0, 1.2, I)      (2.0, 2.1, D)

                                        3   1   3 2        5 1   1   1 1      3 1     1 2 2      6         1 1 1
    b. Definite radiculopathy           1 2 3 4 5 6 7 8 9  1 2 3 4 5 6 7 8 9  1 2 3 4 5 6 7 8 9  1 2 3 4 5 6 7 8 9   (245-248)
                                          (5.0, 1.8, I)      (1.0, 1.7, I)      (5.0, 2.3, I)      (1.0, 2.0, I)
```

Appropriateness scale: 1 = extremely inappropriate, 5 = uncertain, 9 = extremely appropriate.

```
Chapter 6
CERVICAL SPINAL MANIPULATION OR MOBILIZATION
IS APPROPRIATE WITH:                          NO OTHER ADEQUATE CONSERVATIVE        NONMANIPULATIVE CONSERVATIVE CARE
SUBACUTE OR CHRONIC NECK PAIN AND CLINICAL       CARE FOR THIS EPISODE               FOR THIS EPISODE HAS FAILED
SUSPICION OF CERVICAL NERVE ROOT INVOLVEMENT  -----------------------------------   -----------------------------------
AND                                             Mobilization      Manipulation       Mobilization      Manipulation

NO RADIOGRAPHIC CONTRAINDICATIONS AND

G. Clinically substantial traumatic etiology
   and no previous response to
   prior SMT AND

   1. No advanced imaging studies AND
                                              1 2 1 2 1 1 1     3 3     1 1 1         2 2   3 1 1     4 2     1 1 1
      a. Possible Radiculopathy               1 2 3 4 5 6 7 8 9 1 2 3 4 5 6 7 8 9 1 2 3 4 5 6 7 8 9 1 2 3 4 5 6 7 8 9   (249-252)
                                                (4.0, 1.6, I)     (2.0, 1.7, I)     (5.0, 1.4, I)     (2.0, 1.8, I)

                                              2 3 1   2   1     5 1   1 2         2 2   2 2   1     5 1 1   1   1
      b. Definite radiculopathy               1 2 3 4 5 6 7 8 9 1 2 3 4 5 6 7 8 9 1 2 3 4 5 6 7 8 9 1 2 3 4 5 6 7 8 9   (253-256)
                                                (2.0, 1.6, I)     (1.0, 1.3, I)     (4.0, 1.7, I)     (1.0, 1.4, A)
   2. Advanced imaging studies show no
      abnormalities AND
                                              1       3 1 4       2 1 2   1 2 1       1 1 2   3 2       1 2 2 1   1 2
      a. Possible Radiculopathy               1 2 3 4 5 6 7 8 9 1 2 3 4 5 6 7 8 9 1 2 3 4 5 6 7 8 9 1 2 3 4 5 6 7 8 9   (257-260)
                                                (6.0, 1.2, I)     (4.0, 1.9, D)     (7.0, 1.4, I)     (4.0, 1.8, D)

                                              3     1 1 1 3     3 2     1 1 2     3 1       2 1 2   3 2   1   1 1 1
      b. Definite radiculopathy               1 2 3 4 5 6 7 8 9 1 2 3 4 5 6 7 8 9 1 2 3 4 5 6 7 8 9 1 2 3 4 5 6 7 8 9   (261-264)
                                                (5.0, 2.2, D)     (2.0, 2.2, I)     (6.0, 2.7, D)     (2.0, 2.2, I)
   3. Advanced imaging findings of cervical
      disc herniation AND
                                              2 1 2   2 2       4 1 1   3         2 1 1   3 2       4 2       3
      a. Possible Radiculopathy               1 2 3 4 5 6 7 8 9 1 2 3 4 5 6 7 8 9 1 2 3 4 5 6 7 8 9 1 2 3 4 5 6 7 8 9   (265-268)
                                                (3.0, 1.7, I)     (2.0, 1.6, I)     (5.0, 1.7, I)     (2.0, 1.8, I)

                                              3 1 2 1 2         5 1   2 1         3 2   2   2       6       1 1 1
      b. Definite radiculopathy               1 2 3 4 5 6 7 8 9 1 2 3 4 5 6 7 8 9 1 2 3 4 5 6 7 8 9 1 2 3 4 5 6 7 8 9   (269-272)
                                                (3.0, 1.3, I)     (1.0, 1.2, I)     (2.0, 1.7, I)     (1.0, 1.3, I)
   4. Advanced imaging findings of cervical
      spinal canal stenosis AND
                                              2 2   2 2 1       5 1     2 1       2 2     2 3       4 2       2 1
      a. Possible Radiculopathy               1 2 3 4 5 6 7 8 9 1 2 3 4 5 6 7 8 9 1 2 3 4 5 6 7 8 9 1 2 3 4 5 6 7 8 9   (273-276)
                                                (4.0, 1.6, I)     (1.0, 1.6, I)     (5.0, 1.9, I)     (2.0, 1.9, I)

                                              3 1 1 2 2         5 1 1 1 1         3 1   1 4         5 1 1   1 1
      b. Definite radiculopathy               1 2 3 4 5 6 7 8 9 1 2 3 4 5 6 7 8 9 1 2 3 4 5 6 7 8 9 1 2 3 4 5 6 7 8 9   (277-280)
                                                (3.0, 1.4, I)     (1.0, 1.1, A)     (4.0, 1.7, I)     (1.0, 1.3, A)
   5. Advanced imaging findings of cervical
      spinal foraminal osteophytosis AND
                                              1   1 1 3 3       4   2   1 2       1   1 1 2 3 1     3   3     1 2
      a. Possible Radiculopathy               1 2 3 4 5 6 7 8 9 1 2 3 4 5 6 7 8 9 1 2 3 4 5 6 7 8 9 1 2 3 4 5 6 7 8 9   (281-284)
                                                (5.0, 1.1, A)     (3.0, 1.8, I)     (5.0, 1.3, I)     (3.0, 1.9, I)

                                              3   1 1 3 1       5 1   1 1 1       3 1     3 2       5 1       3
      b. Definite radiculopathy               1 2 3 4 5 6 7 8 9 1 2 3 4 5 6 7 8 9 1 2 3 4 5 6 7 8 9 1 2 3 4 5 6 7 8 9   (285-288)
                                                (4.0, 1.7, I)     (1.0, 1.4, I)     (5.0, 1.9, I)     (1.0, 1.8, I)
```

Appropriateness scale: 1 = extremely inappropriate, 5 = uncertain, 9 = extremely appropriate.

Chapter 6 CERVICAL SPINAL MANIPULATION OR MOBILIZATION IS APPROPRIATE WITH: SUBACUTE OR CHRONIC NECK PAIN AND CLINICAL SUSPICION OF CERVICAL NERVE ROOT INVOLVEMENT AND	NO OTHER ADEQUATE CONSERVATIVE CARE FOR THIS EPISODE Mobilization	 Manipulation	NONMANIPULATIVE CONSERVATIVE CARE FOR THIS EPISODE HAS FAILED Mobilization	 Manipulation	
H. Clinically substantial traumatic etiology and unfavorable previous response to prior SMT AND					
1. No advanced imaging studies AND					
a. Possible Radiculopathy	3 1 2 1 1 1 1 2 3 4 5 6 7 8 9 (3.0, 1.4, I)	6 1 2 1 2 3 4 5 6 7 8 9 (1.0, 1.0, A)	2 1 1 3 1 1 1 2 3 4 5 6 7 8 9 (4.0, 1.3, I)	5 2 2 1 2 3 4 5 6 7 8 9 (1.0, 1.1, A)	(289-292)
b. Definite radiculopathy	4 2 2 1 1 2 3 4 5 6 7 8 9 (2.0, 1.3, I)	7 1 1 1 2 3 4 5 6 7 8 9 (1.0, 0.6, A)	3 1 2 2 1 1 2 3 4 5 6 7 8 9 (3.0, 1.3, I)	7 1 1 1 2 3 4 5 6 7 8 9 (1.0, 0.8, A)	(293-296)
2. Advanced imaging studies show no abnormalities AND					
a. Possible Radiculopathy	1 1 2 2 3 1 2 3 4 5 6 7 8 9 (5.0, 1.6, I)	4 1 1 2 1 1 2 3 4 5 6 7 8 9 (2.0, 1.9, I)	1 1 2 1 2 2 1 2 3 4 5 6 7 8 9 (5.0, 1.9, I)	4 1 2 1 1 1 2 3 4 5 6 7 8 9 (3.0, 1.9, I)	(297-300)
b. Definite radiculopathy	3 1 1 2 2 1 2 3 4 5 6 7 8 9 (4.0, 1.9, I)	5 1 1 1 1 1 2 3 4 5 6 7 8 9 (1.0, 1.4, I)	4 3 1 1 1 2 3 4 5 6 7 8 9 (5.0, 2.1, I)	5 2 2 1 2 3 4 5 6 7 8 9 (1.0, 1.6, A)	(301-304)
3. Advanced imaging findings of cervical disc herniation AND					
a. Possible Radiculopathy	3 2 2 2 1 2 3 4 5 6 7 8 9 (2.0, 1.4, I)	6 2 1 1 2 3 4 5 6 7 8 9 (1.0, 0.8, A)	3 1 1 2 2 1 2 3 4 5 6 7 8 9 (3.0, 1.4, I)	6 1 1 1 1 2 3 4 5 6 7 8 9 (1.0, 1.0, A)	(305-308)
b. Definite radiculopathy	4 2 1 2 1 2 3 4 5 6 7 8 9 (2.0, 1.0, A)	7 2 1 2 3 4 5 6 7 8 9 (1.0, 0.4, A)	5 2 2 1 2 3 4 5 6 7 8 9 (1.0, 1.3, A)	6 1 2 1 2 3 4 5 6 7 8 9 (1.0, 0.8, A)	(309-312)
4. Advanced imaging findings of cervical spinal canal stenosis AND					
a. Possible Radiculopathy	3 1 2 2 1 1 2 3 4 5 6 7 8 9 (3.0, 1.2, I)	6 2 1 1 2 3 4 5 6 7 8 9 (1.0, 0.9, A)	3 1 2 3 1 2 3 4 5 6 7 8 9 (4.0, 1.6, I)	6 2 1 1 2 3 4 5 6 7 8 9 (1.0, 1.2, I)	(313-316)
b. Definite radiculopathy	4 1 2 2 1 2 3 4 5 6 7 8 9 (2.0, 1.1, A)	7 1 1 1 2 3 4 5 6 7 8 9 (1.0, 0.4, A)	4 1 4 1 2 3 4 5 6 7 8 9 (3.0, 1.3, I)	7 1 1 1 2 3 4 5 6 7 8 9 (1.0, 0.7, A)	(317-320)
5. Advanced imaging findings of cervical spinal foraminal osteophytosis AND					
a. Possible Radiculopathy	1 3 3 2 1 2 3 4 5 6 7 8 9 (4.0, 1.2, I)	6 1 1 1 1 2 3 4 5 6 7 8 9 (1.0, 0.9, A)	1 3 1 3 1 1 2 3 4 5 6 7 8 9 (4.0, 1.6, I)	5 1 2 1 1 2 3 4 5 6 7 8 9 (1.0, 1.3, I)	(321-324)
b. Definite radiculopathy	4 1 3 1 1 2 3 4 5 6 7 8 9 (3.0, 1.4, I)	7 2 1 2 3 4 5 6 7 8 9 (1.0, 0.7, A)	4 3 2 1 2 3 4 5 6 7 8 9 (4.0, 1.6, I)	6 1 1 1 1 2 3 4 5 6 7 8 9 (1.0, 1.0, A)	(325-328)

Appropriateness scale: 1 = extremely inappropriate, 5 = uncertain, 9 = extremely appropriate.

```
Chapter 7
CERVICAL SPINAL MANIPULATION OR MOBILIZATION
IS APPROPRIATE WITH:
GENERALIZED NECK PAIN WITH NO CLINICAL
SUSPICION OF CONNECTIVE TISSUE DISEASE AND       Mobilization         Manipulation

A. Morning stiffness in the neck AND

 1. Radiographic findings of early
    degenerative changes in the cervical
    spine AND
                                                    6 3                6 2   1
    a. No prior care for this condition     1 2 3 4 5 6 7 8 9   1 2 3 4 5 6 7 8 9          (  1-  2)
                                              (7.0, 0.3, A)       (6.0, 0.6, I)

    b. Non-manipulative care for this               3 6                2 4 2 1
       condition has not helped             1 2 3 4 5 6 7 8 9   1 2 3 4 5 6 7 8 9          (  3-  4)
                                              (8.0, 0.3, A)       (7.0, 0.7, A)
 2. Radiographic findings of moderate
    degeneration in the cervical spine AND
                                                  1 7 1              2 5 1 1
    a. No prior care for this condition     1 2 3 4 5 6 7 8 9   1 2 3 4 5 6 7 8 9          (  5-  6)
                                              (7.0, 0.2, A)       (6.0, 0.6, A)

    b. Non-manipulative care for this             2 1 6              3   3 2 1
       condition has not helped             1 2 3 4 5 6 7 8 9   1 2 3 4 5 6 7 8 9          (  7-  8)
                                              (8.0, 0.6, A)       (7.0, 1.1, I)
 3. Radiographic findings of advanced
    degeneration in the cervical spine AND
                                                  8 1           1   2 5   1
    a. No prior care for this condition     1 2 3 4 5 6 7 8 9   1 2 3 4 5 6 7 8 9          (  9- 10)
                                              (6.0, 0.1, A)       (5.0, 0.8, A)

    b. Non-manipulative care for this           1 1 7           1   2 2 2 1 1
       condition has not helped             1 2 3 4 5 6 7 8 9   1 2 3 4 5 6 7 8 9          ( 11- 12)
                                              (7.0, 0.3, A)       (5.0, 1.3, I)
```

Appropriateness scale: 1 = extremely inappropriate, 5 = uncertain, 9 = extremely appropriate.

```
Chapter 7
CERVICAL SPINAL MANIPULATION OR MOBILIZATION
IS APPROPRIATE WITH:
GENERALIZED NECK PAIN WITH NO CLINICAL
SUSPICION OF CONNECTIVE TISSUE DISEASE AND     Mobilization       Manipulation

B. Morning pain and stiffness in the neck and
   periodic flare-up of symptoms with diffuse
   non-radicular referred pain AND

   1. Radiographic findings of early
      degenerative changes in the cervical
      spine AND
                                                         2 5 2            2 5 1   1
      a. No prior care for this condition       1 2 3 4 5 6 7 8 9  1 2 3 4 5 6 7 8 9     ( 13- 14)
                                                 (7.0, 0.4, A)      (6.0, 0.7, A)

      b. Non-manipulative care for this                1   3 5          1 1 1 4 1 1
         condition has not helped               1 2 3 4 5 6 7 8 9  1 2 3 4 5 6 7 8 9     ( 15- 16)
                                                 (8.0, 0.7, A)      (7.0, 1.0, I)
   2. Radiographic findings of moderate
      degeneration in the cervical spine AND
                                                       1   8            1 1 5 1 1
      a. No prior care for this condition       1 2 3 4 5 6 7 8 9  1 2 3 4 5 6 7 8 9     ( 17- 18)
                                                 (7.0, 0.2, A)      (6.0, 0.7, A)

      b. Non-manipulative care for this              1     4 4          2   2 3 1 1
         condition has not helped               1 2 3 4 5 6 7 8 9  1 2 3 4 5 6 7 8 9     ( 19- 20)
                                                 (7.0, 0.8, A)      (7.0, 1.2, I)
   3. Radiographic findings of advanced
      degeneration in the cervical spine AND
                                                       1 6 2          1 3 4   1
      a. No prior care for this condition       1 2 3 4 5 6 7 8 9  1 2 3 4 5 6 7 8 9     ( 21- 22)
                                                 (6.0, 0.3, A)      (5.0, 0.8, A)

      b. Non-manipulative care for this              1   2 6          2 1 2 3   1
         condition has not helped               1 2 3 4 5 6 7 8 9  1 2 3 4 5 6 7 8 9     ( 23- 24)
                                                 (7.0, 0.6, I)      (5.0, 1.2, I)
```

Appropriateness scale: 1 = extremely inappropriate, 5 = uncertain, 9 = extremely appropriate.

Chapter 8 CERVICAL SPINAL MANIPULATION OR MOBILIZATION IS INDICATED FOR A PATIENT WITH: ACUTE, CONSTANT HEADACE	NO OTHER ADEQUATE CONSERVATIVE CARE FOR THIS EPISODE		NONMANIPULATIVE CONSERVATIVE CARE FOR THIS EPISODE HAS FAILED		
	Mobilization	Manipulation	Mobilization	Manipulation	
ACUTE, SUDDEN, CONSTANT, PERSISTANT HEADACHE, WITHOUT HISTORY OF RELATED CERVICAL SPINE TRAUMA	9 1 2 3 4 5 6 7 8 9 (1.0, 0.0, A)	9 1 2 3 4 5 6 7 8 9 (1.0, 0.0, A)	9 1 2 3 4 5 6 7 8 9 (1.0, 0.0, A)	9 1 2 3 4 5 6 7 8 9 (1.0, 0.0, A)	(1- 4)

Appropriateness scale: 1 = extremely inappropriate, 5 = uncertain, 9 = extremely appropriate.

Chapter 8 CERVICAL SPINAL MANIPULATION OR MOBILIZATION IS INDICATED FOR A PATIENT WITH: ACUTE, CONSTANT HEADACE	NO OTHER ADEQUATE CONSERVATIVE CARE FOR THIS EPISODE		NONMANIPULATIVE CONSERVATIVE CARE FOR THIS EPISODE HAS FAILED		
	Mobilization	Manipulation	Mobilization	Manipulation	
HISTORY OF RELATED CERVICAL SPINE TRAUMA					
NO CERVICAL SPINE RADIOGRAPHS	9 1 2 3 4 5 6 7 8 9 (1.0, 0.0, A)	9 1 2 3 4 5 6 7 8 9 (1.0, 0.0, A)	9 1 2 3 4 5 6 7 8 9 (1.0, 0.0, A)	9 1 2 3 4 5 6 7 8 9 (1.0, 0.0, A)	(5- 8)
NO RADIOGRAPHIC CONTRAINDICATIONS AND					
1. No neurologic findings or post-traumatic neurologic symptoms AND					
a. Cervical signs and/or symptoms AND					
- no prior SMT	1 5 2 1 2 3 4 5 6 7 8 9 (6.0, 0.6, I)	1 3 2 1 1 1 2 3 4 5 6 7 8 9 (5.5, 1.4, I)	2 4 2 1 2 3 4 5 6 7 8 9 (7.0, 0.8, A)	1 2 1 3 1 1 2 3 4 5 6 7 8 9 (6.5, 1.5, I)	(9- 12)
- favorable experience with prior SMT	1 2 5 1 1 2 3 4 5 6 7 8 9 (7.0, 0.7, I)	1 5 2 1 1 2 3 4 5 6 7 8 9 (6.0, 1.0, I)	2 2 5 1 2 3 4 5 6 7 8 9 (8.0, 0.7, A)	1 3 2 2 1 1 2 3 4 5 6 7 8 9 (7.0, 1.1, I)	(13- 16)
- no response to prior SMT	1 1 1 5 1 1 2 3 4 5 6 7 8 9 (6.0, 0.8, A)	1 1 2 1 2 1 1 1 2 3 4 5 6 7 8 9 (5.0, 1.7, I)	1 1 5 2 1 2 3 4 5 6 7 8 9 (6.0, 0.6, A)	1 1 2 1 2 1 1 1 2 3 4 5 6 7 8 9 (5.0, 1.6, I)	(17- 20)
- unfavorable response to prior SMT	5 3 1 1 2 3 4 5 6 7 8 9 (3.0, 1.0, I)	2 1 3 1 1 1 1 2 3 4 5 6 7 8 9 (3.0, 1.3, I)	1 2 4 2 1 2 3 4 5 6 7 8 9 (5.0, 1.0, I)	1 3 3 1 1 1 2 3 4 5 6 7 8 9 (4.0, 1.4, I)	(21- 24)
b. No cervical signs and/or symptoms AND					
- no prior SMT	3 2 1 3 1 2 3 4 5 6 7 8 9 (4.0, 1.1, I)	2 1 1 4 1 1 2 3 4 5 6 7 8 9 (5.0, 1.6, I)	1 4 4 1 2 3 4 5 6 7 8 9 (5.0, 0.7, A)	2 1 2 3 1 1 2 3 4 5 6 7 8 9 (5.0, 1.4, I)	(25- 28)
- favorable experience with prior SMT	2 1 2 2 2 1 2 3 4 5 6 7 8 9 (5.0, 1.2, I)	1 1 1 1 4 1 1 2 3 4 5 6 7 8 9 (6.0, 1.3, I)	1 1 2 5 1 2 3 4 5 6 7 8 9 (7.0, 0.9, I)	1 2 2 4 1 2 3 4 5 6 7 8 9 (6.0, 1.0, I)	(29- 32)
- no response to prior SMT	3 4 2 1 2 3 4 5 6 7 8 9 (4.0, 0.6, I)	1 3 2 2 1 1 2 3 4 5 6 7 8 9 (3.0, 1.0, I)	1 1 5 2 1 2 3 4 5 6 7 8 9 (5.0, 0.6, A)	2 2 3 1 1 1 2 3 4 5 6 7 8 9 (4.0, 1.0, I)	(33- 36)
- unfavorable response to prior SMT	2 3 3 1 1 2 3 4 5 6 7 8 9 (2.0, 0.8, A)	5 2 1 1 1 2 3 4 5 6 7 8 9 (1.0, 0.8, A)	2 1 1 3 2 1 2 3 4 5 6 7 8 9 (4.0, 1.2, I)	3 2 3 1 1 2 3 4 5 6 7 8 9 (2.0, 1.0, A)	(37- 40)

Appropriateness scale: 1 = extremely inappropriate, 5 = uncertain, 9 = extremely appropriate.

```
Chapter 8                                    NO OTHER ADEQUATE CONSERVATIVE        NONMANIPULATIVE CONSERVATIVE CARE
CERVICAL SPINAL MANIPULATION OR MOBILIZATION      CARE FOR THIS EPISODE             FOR THIS EPISODE HAS FAILED
IS INDICATED FOR A PATIENT WITH:             -----------------------------------  -----------------------------------
ACUTE, CONSTANT HEADACE                         Mobilization       Manipulation      Mobilization       Manipulation

  2. No neurologic findings and mild
     post-traumatic neurologic symptoms AND

     a. Cervical signs and/or symptoms AND
                                                  2   2 3 2      1 1   4   1 1   1          2 2 2 1 2    2   4       2 1
        - no prior SMT                       1 2 3 4 5 6 7 8 9  1 2 3 4 5 6 7 8 9  1 2 3 4 5 6 7 8 9  1 2 3 4 5 6 7 8 9      ( 41- 44)
                                               (6.0, 1.1, I)      (4.0, 1.7, I)      (6.0, 1.2, I)      (4.0, 1.7, I)

        - favorable experience with                2   3 3 1    1   1   3 2 1   1            2 1 4 2        2 4   2   1
          prior SMT                          1 2 3 4 5 6 7 8 9  1 2 3 4 5 6 7 8 9  1 2 3 4 5 6 7 8 9  1 2 3 4 5 6 7 8 9      ( 45- 48)
                                               (6.0, 1.0, I)      (5.0, 1.6, I)      (7.0, 0.8, I)      (5.0, 1.1, I)

                                                 3   3 2 1      2 2 1 1   1 1 1      1 1   4 1 2          2 2 1 1 1 1 1
        - no response to prior SMT           1 2 3 4 5 6 7 8 9  1 2 3 4 5 6 7 8 9  1 2 3 4 5 6 7 8 9  1 2 3 4 5 6 7 8 9      ( 49- 52)
                                               (5.0, 1.1, I)      (3.0, 2.1, I)      (5.0, 1.1, I)      (4.0, 1.8, I)

                                             1 1 3 1 2 1        5 1 1   1   1      2   1 2 2 2        3 1   3 1   1
        - unfavorable response to prior SMT  1 2 3 4 5 6 7 8 9  1 2 3 4 5 6 7 8 9  1 2 3 4 5 6 7 8 9  1 2 3 4 5 6 7 8 9      ( 53- 56)
                                               (3.0, 1.2, I)      (1.0, 1.4, A)      (4.0, 1.4, I)      (4.0, 1.7, I)
     b. No cervical signs and/or symptoms
        AND
                                             1   4 1 2 1        2 4 1   1 1        1 1   2 3 2        1 4 1       2 1
        - no prior SMT                       1 2 3 4 5 6 7 8 9  1 2 3 4 5 6 7 8 9  1 2 3 4 5 6 7 8 9  1 2 3 4 5 6 7 8 9      ( 57- 60)
                                               (3.0, 1.1, I)      (2.0, 1.1, A)      (5.0, 1.2, A)      (2.0, 1.7, I)

        - favorable experience with            1 2 3   2 1      2   4   1 1 1          2   2 4 1      1   2 2 1 1 2
          prior SMT                          1 2 3 4 5 6 7 8 9  1 2 3 4 5 6 7 8 9  1 2 3 4 5 6 7 8 9  1 2 3 4 5 6 7 8 9      ( 61- 64)
                                               (4.0, 1.2, I)      (3.0, 1.4, I)      (6.0, 1.0, I)      (4.0, 1.6, I)

                                             1   4 3 1          3 3 1 1 1          1 3 1 1 2 1        2 3 1 2   1
        - no response to prior SMT           1 2 3 4 5 6 7 8 9  1 2 3 4 5 6 7 8 9  1 2 3 4 5 6 7 8 9  1 2 3 4 5 6 7 8 9      ( 65- 68)
                                               (3.0, 0.8, I)      (2.0, 1.0, A)      (3.0, 1.4, I)      (2.0, 1.2, I)

                                             3 1 5              6 2   1            3 3   2 1          5 3     1
        - unfavorable response to prior SMT  1 2 3 4 5 6 7 8 9  1 2 3 4 5 6 7 8 9  1 2 3 4 5 6 7 8 9  1 2 3 4 5 6 7 8 9      ( 69- 72)
                                               (3.0, 0.8, A)      (1.0, 0.6, A)      (2.0, 1.1, I)      (1.0, 0.8, A)

                                             9                  9                  9                  9
  3. Any new focal neurologic findings       1 2 3 4 5 6 7 8 9  1 2 3 4 5 6 7 8 9  1 2 3 4 5 6 7 8 9  1 2 3 4 5 6 7 8 9      ( 73- 76)
                                               (1.0, 0.0, A)      (1.0, 0.0, A)      (1.0, 0.0, A)      (1.0, 0.0, A)
```

Appropriateness scale: 1 = extremely inappropriate, 5 = uncertain, 9 = extremely appropriate.

```
Chapter 9                                     NO OTHER ADEQUATE CONSERVATIVE       NONMANIPULATIVE CONSERVATIVE CARE
CERVICAL SPINAL MANIPULATION OR MOBILIZATION     CARE FOR THIS EPISODE              FOR THIS EPISODE HAS FAILED
IS INDICATED FOR A PATIENT WITH:              -----------------------------------  -----------------------------------
ACUTE OR SUBACUTE INTERMITTENT HEADACHE AND     Mobilization      Manipulation       Mobilization      Manipulation

                                                    3 1 4       1 2 1   2 1 1                 3 2 3   1 1   1 1 2 1 1
NO CERVICAL SPINE RADIOGRAPHS                 1 2 3 4 5 6 7 8 9 1 2 3 4 5 6 7 8 9 1 2 3 4 5 6 7 8 9 1 2 3 4 5 6 7 8 9   (  1-  4)
                                               (5.5, 0.9, A)     (4.0, 1.9, I)     (6.0, 0.8, I)     (5.5, 1.9, I)

NO RADIOGRAPHIC CONTRAINDICATIONS AND

A. No history of related cervical spine
   trauma AND

  1. No neurologic symptoms or findings AND

    a. Cervical signs and/or symptoms AND
                                                  1       6 1 1   1     3   3   2             6 2 1       1 2 1 1 2 2
      - no prior SMT                          1 2 3 4 5 6 7 8 9 1 2 3 4 5 6 7 8 9 1 2 3 4 5 6 7 8 9 1 2 3 4 5 6 7 8 9   (  5-  8)
                                               (7.0, 0.8, A)     (7.0, 1.7, I)     (7.0, 0.4, A)     (7.0, 1.6, I)

      - favorable experience with                 1       3 3 2   1       3   2 3             3 4 2         1 1 2 1 4
        prior SMT                             1 2 3 4 5 6 7 8 9 1 2 3 4 5 6 7 8 9 1 2 3 4 5 6 7 8 9 1 2 3 4 5 6 7 8 9   (  9- 12)
                                               (8.0, 1.1, A)     (8.0, 1.7, I)     (8.0, 0.6, A)     (8.0, 1.2, A)

                                                  1   4 1 3       1 2 1 1 1 3       1   1 1 4 2       1 2   2   3 1
      - no response to prior SMT              1 2 3 4 5 6 7 8 9 1 2 3 4 5 6 7 8 9 1 2 3 4 5 6 7 8 9 1 2 3 4 5 6 7 8 9   ( 13- 16)
                                               (5.0, 1.0, I)     (5.0, 1.7, D)     (6.0, 1.0, I)     (5.0, 1.8, D)

                                              1 1 1 3 2 1       2 1 3 1 1 1       1 2 1   4 1       2 2   2 2   1
      - unfavorable response to prior SMT     1 2 3 4 5 6 7 8 9 1 2 3 4 5 6 7 8 9 1 2 3 4 5 6 7 8 9 1 2 3 4 5 6 7 8 9   ( 17- 20)
                                               (4.0, 1.1, I)     (3.0, 1.2, I)     (5.0, 1.4, I)     (4.0, 1.7, I)
    b. No cervical signs and/or symptoms
       AND
                                                1     5 3       1   3   3 1   1       1   2 5 1     1 1 3 1 2     1
      - no prior SMT                          1 2 3 4 5 6 7 8 9 1 2 3 4 5 6 7 8 9 1 2 3 4 5 6 7 8 9 1 2 3 4 5 6 7 8 9   ( 21- 24)
                                               (5.0, 0.7, A)     (5.0, 1.6, I)     (6.0, 0.7, A)     (4.0, 1.3, I)

      - favorable experience with                 1   2 2 3 1     1 1 1 1 2 1 2       1     2 4 2     1     3 1 2 2
        prior SMT                             1 2 3 4 5 6 7 8 9 1 2 3 4 5 6 7 8 9 1 2 3 4 5 6 7 8 9 1 2 3 4 5 6 7 8 9   ( 25- 28)
                                               (6.0, 1.1, I)     (6.0, 1.7, I)     (7.0, 0.9, I)     (6.0, 1.4, I)

                                                1   6 1 1       1 2 1 2 2 1           1 4 2 2       1 1 3     2 2
      - no response to prior SMT              1 2 3 4 5 6 7 8 9 1 2 3 4 5 6 7 8 9 1 2 3 4 5 6 7 8 9 1 2 3 4 5 6 7 8 9   ( 29- 32)
                                               (4.0, 0.6, A)     (4.0, 1.3, I)     (4.0, 0.8, A)     (3.0, 1.4, I)

                                              1 3 4 1           4 3 1   1         1 2 3 2 1         4 2 1 1 1
      - unfavorable response to prior SMT     1 2 3 4 5 6 7 8 9 1 2 3 4 5 6 7 8 9 1 2 3 4 5 6 7 8 9 1 2 3 4 5 6 7 8 9   ( 33- 36)
                                               (3.0, 0.7, A)     (2.0, 0.9, A)     (3.0, 0.9, I)     (2.0, 1.1, A)
```

Appropriateness scale: 1 = extremely inappropriate, 5 = uncertain, 9 = extremely appropriate.

```
Chapter 9                                     NO OTHER ADEQUATE CONSERVATIVE        NONMANIPULATIVE CONSERVATIVE CARE
CERVICAL SPINAL MANIPULATION OR MOBILIZATION    CARE FOR THIS EPISODE                 FOR THIS EPISODE HAS FAILED
IS INDICATED FOR A PATIENT WITH:              ------------------------------------  ------------------------------------
ACUTE OR SUBACUTE INTERMITTENT HEADACHE AND     Mobilization       Manipulation       Mobilization       Manipulation

  2. Mild post-traumatic-like neuologic
     symptoms and a normal neurologic exam
     AND

     a. Cervical signs and/or symptoms AND
                                                  1       4 3 1  1   2 1 1 1 1 1 1      1   1 2 3 1 1  1 2 1 2       1 2
        - no prior SMT                            1 2 3 4 5 6 7 8 9  1 2 3 4 5 6 7 8 9  1 2 3 4 5 6 7 8 9  1 2 3 4 5 6 7 8 9   ( 37- 40)
                                                   (6.0, 0.9, I)      (5.0, 2.1, D)      (7.0, 1.2, I)      (5.0, 2.1, D)

        - favorable experience with                   1       5 2 1  1     1   3   2 2      1       3 4 1    1     2 1 2   3
          prior SMT                               1 2 3 4 5 6 7 8 9  1 2 3 4 5 6 7 8 9  1 2 3 4 5 6 7 8 9  1 2 3 4 5 6 7 8 9   ( 41- 44)
                                                   (7.0, 0.9, A)      (6.0, 1.9, I)      (8.0, 1.0, A)      (7.0, 1.8, I)

                                                    1   3 3   2      1 2 2   2   2        1   1 3 3 1      1 1 3   1   2 1
        - no response to prior SMT                1 2 3 4 5 6 7 8 9  1 2 3 4 5 6 7 8 9  1 2 3 4 5 6 7 8 9  1 2 3 4 5 6 7 8 9   ( 45- 48)
                                                   (5.0, 1.1, I)      (3.0, 1.8, I)      (5.0, 1.0, A)      (3.0, 2.0, D)

                                                  1 2 2 3   1        4 2 1   1 1        1 2 2 1 2 1        4 2     2   1
        - unfavorable response to prior SMT       1 2 3 4 5 6 7 8 9  1 2 3 4 5 6 7 8 9  1 2 3 4 5 6 7 8 9  1 2 3 4 5 6 7 8 9   ( 49- 52)
                                                   (3.0, 1.1, I)      (2.0, 1.3, A)      (3.0, 1.3, I)      (2.0, 1.7, I)
     b. No cervical signs and/or symptoms
        AND
                                                    1   2 4 2        2 1 2 1 1 1   1      1 1 1 1 4 1      2 1 1 1 1 2   1
        - no prior SMT                            1 2 3 4 5 6 7 8 9  1 2 3 4 5 6 7 8 9  1 2 3 4 5 6 7 8 9  1 2 3 4 5 6 7 8 9   ( 53- 56)
                                                   (5.0, 0.8, A)      (3.0, 1.8, I)      (6.0, 1.2, I)      (4.0, 2.0, I)

        - favorable experience with                 1     2 3 3      1   2 1 1 2 1 1          1 1 2 5        1 1 3 1   2 1
          prior SMT                               1 2 3 4 5 6 7 8 9  1 2 3 4 5 6 7 8 9  1 2 3 4 5 6 7 8 9  1 2 3 4 5 6 7 8 9   ( 57- 60)
                                                   (6.0, 1.0, I)      (5.0, 1.8, I)      (7.0, 0.8, I)      (4.0, 1.6, I)

                                                  1   1 5 1 1        1 3 1 1 2 1        1 1   2 3 2        1 3   1 2 2
        - no response to prior SMT                1 2 3 4 5 6 7 8 9  1 2 3 4 5 6 7 8 9  1 2 3 4 5 6 7 8 9  1 2 3 4 5 6 7 8 9   ( 61- 64)
                                                   (4.0, 0.8, A)      (3.0, 1.4, I)      (5.0, 1.2, A)      (4.0, 1.7, I)

                                                  2 2 4 1            5 1 2   1          3 2 1 2 1          5 1 1 1 1
        - unfavorable response to prior SMT       1 2 3 4 5 6 7 8 9  1 2 3 4 5 6 7 8 9  1 2 3 4 5 6 7 8 9  1 2 3 4 5 6 7 8 9   ( 65- 68)
                                                   (3.0, 0.8, A)      (1.0, 1.0, A)      (2.0, 1.2, I)      (1.0, 1.1, A)
```

Appropriateness scale: 1 = extremely inappropriate, 5 = uncertain, 9 = extremely appropriate.

```
Chapter 9                                   NO OTHER ADEQUATE CONSERVATIVE        NONMANIPULATIVE CONSERVATIVE CARE
CERVICAL SPINAL MANIPULATION OR MOBILIZATION      CARE FOR THIS EPISODE            FOR THIS EPISODE HAS FAILED
IS INDICATED FOR A PATIENT WITH:            ------------------------------------  ------------------------------------
ACUTE OR SUBACUTE INTERMITTENT HEADACHE AND   Mobilization       Manipulation       Mobilization       Manipulation

NO RADIOGRAPHIC CONTRAINDICATIONS AND

B. History of related cervical spine trauma
   AND

   1. No neurologic symptoms or findings AND

      a. Cervical signs and/or symptoms AND
                                              1     7   1    1     2 3 1   2            2 4 2 1          3 2 2   2
         - no prior SMT                 1 2 3 4 5 6 7 8 9  1 2 3 4 5 6 7 8 9  1 2 3 4 5 6 7 8 9  1 2 3 4 5 6 7 8 9    ( 69- 72)
                                          (7.0, 0.6, A)      (6.0, 1.4, I)      (7.0, 0.7, A)      (6.0, 1.2, I)

                                                1   2 4 2      1     2 1 3 2            1 1 6 1          1 2 1 3 2
         - favorable experience with    1 2 3 4 5 6 7 8 9  1 2 3 4 5 6 7 8 9  1 2 3 4 5 6 7 8 9  1 2 3 4 5 6 7 8 9    ( 73- 76)
           prior SMT                      (8.0, 0.8, A)      (8.0, 1.3, I)      (8.0, 0.4, A)      (8.0, 1.1, I)

                                            1 1 3 2 2      1 1 1   4   2            1 3 2 3        2   2 1 2 1 1
         - no response to prior SMT     1 2 3 4 5 6 7 8 9  1 2 3 4 5 6 7 8 9  1 2 3 4 5 6 7 8 9  1 2 3 4 5 6 7 8 9    ( 77- 80)
                                          (5.0, 1.0, I)      (5.0, 1.4, I)      (6.0, 0.9, I)      (5.0, 1.7, I)

                                        2   2 3 1 1        3 1 2 1 1 1        1 1 1 2 3 1        1 4   1 2   1
         - unfavorable response to prior SMT
                                        1 2 3 4 5 6 7 8 9  1 2 3 4 5 6 7 8 9  1 2 3 4 5 6 7 8 9  1 2 3 4 5 6 7 8 9    ( 81- 84)
                                          (4.0, 1.2, I)      (3.0, 1.4, I)      (4.0, 1.2, I)      (2.0, 1.6, I)
      b. No cervical signs and/or symptoms
         AND
                                            2 1 4 2        1 1 2 3   1   1            2 2 3 2          1 1 2 2 1 1 1
         - no prior SMT                 1 2 3 4 5 6 7 8 9  1 2 3 4 5 6 7 8 9  1 2 3 4 5 6 7 8 9  1 2 3 4 5 6 7 8 9    ( 85- 88)
                                          (5.0, 0.8, A)      (4.0, 1.4, I)      (6.0, 0.9, A)      (5.0, 1.4, I)

                                              2 2 2 3      1       4 2 1 1            1 2   6              4 2 2 1
         - favorable experience with    1 2 3 4 5 6 7 8 9  1 2 3 4 5 6 7 8 9  1 2 3 4 5 6 7 8 9  1 2 3 4 5 6 7 8 9    ( 89- 92)
           prior SMT                      (6.0, 1.0, I)      (5.0, 1.2, I)      (7.0, 0.8, I)      (6.0, 0.9, I)

                                            3 3 3          1 1 3 2 1 1            3   5 1          1 1 1 3 2 1
         - no response to prior SMT     1 2 3 4 5 6 7 8 9  1 2 3 4 5 6 7 8 9  1 2 3 4 5 6 7 8 9  1 2 3 4 5 6 7 8 9    ( 93- 96)
                                          (4.0, 0.7, I)      (3.0, 1.1, I)      (5.0, 0.8, I)      (4.0, 1.1, I)

                                        2 3 3 1            4 3 1   1          2 3 1 3            4 2 2   1
         - unfavorable response to prior SMT
                                        1 2 3 4 5 6 7 8 9  1 2 3 4 5 6 7 8 9  1 2 3 4 5 6 7 8 9  1 2 3 4 5 6 7 8 9    ( 97-100)
                                          (2.0, 0.8, A)      (2.0, 0.9, A)      (2.0, 1.0, I)      (2.0, 1.0, A)
```

Appropriateness scale: 1 = extremely inappropriate, 5 = uncertain, 9 = extremely appropriate.

Chapter 9 CERVICAL SPINAL MANIPULATION OR MOBILIZATION IS INDICATED FOR A PATIENT WITH: ACUTE OR SUBACUTE INTERMITTENT HEADACHE AND	NO OTHER ADEQUATE CONSERVATIVE CARE FOR THIS EPISODE Mobilization	NO OTHER ADEQUATE CONSERVATIVE CARE FOR THIS EPISODE Manipulation	NONMANIPULATIVE CONSERVATIVE CARE FOR THIS EPISODE HAS FAILED Mobilization	NONMANIPULATIVE CONSERVATIVE CARE FOR THIS EPISODE HAS FAILED Manipulation	
2. Mild post-traumatic-like neuologic symptoms and a normal neurologic exam AND					
a. Cervical signs and/or symptoms AND					
- no prior SMT	1 1 3 3 1 1 2 3 4 5 6 7 8 9 (6.0, 1.1, I)	1 1 2 2 1 2 1 2 3 4 5 6 7 8 9 (5.0, 2.0, I)	2 2 3 1 1 1 2 3 4 5 6 7 8 9 (7.0, 1.0, I)	2 1 3 1 2 1 2 3 4 5 6 7 8 9 (5.0, 2.0, D)	(101-104)
- favorable experience with prior SMT	1 6 1 1 1 2 3 4 5 6 7 8 9 (7.0, 0.7, A)	1 3 1 1 1 2 1 2 3 4 5 6 7 8 9 (6.0, 1.8, I)	1 4 3 1 1 2 3 4 5 6 7 8 9 (7.0, 0.9, A)	1 2 3 1 2 1 2 3 4 5 6 7 8 9 (6.0, 1.6, I)	(105-108)
- no response to prior SMT	1 6 1 1 1 2 3 4 5 6 7 8 9 (5.0, 0.8, A)	1 2 3 1 2 1 2 3 4 5 6 7 8 9 (4.0, 1.6, I)	1 4 3 1 1 2 3 4 5 6 7 8 9 (5.0, 0.7, A)	2 1 2 1 1 1 1 1 2 3 4 5 6 7 8 9 (4.0, 1.7, I)	(109-112)
- unfavorable response to prior SMT	2 2 1 3 1 1 2 3 4 5 6 7 8 9 (3.0, 1.3, I)	5 1 1 1 1 1 2 3 4 5 6 7 8 9 (1.0, 1.3, A)	1 1 3 1 2 1 1 2 3 4 5 6 7 8 9 (3.0, 1.2, I)	4 2 1 1 1 1 2 3 4 5 6 7 8 9 (2.0, 1.6, I)	(113-116)
b. No cervical signs and/or symptoms AND					
- no prior SMT	3 1 3 2 1 2 3 4 5 6 7 8 9 (5.0, 1.0, I)	1 2 2 2 1 1 1 2 3 4 5 6 7 8 9 (3.0, 1.6, I)	2 2 1 2 2 1 2 3 4 5 6 7 8 9 (5.0, 1.3, I)	2 3 2 1 1 1 2 3 4 5 6 7 8 9 (3.0, 1.4, I)	(117-120)
- favorable experience with prior SMT	4 3 2 1 2 3 4 5 6 7 8 9 (6.0, 0.7, A)	1 2 1 1 2 1 1 1 2 3 4 5 6 7 8 9 (5.0, 1.8, I)	2 1 1 5 1 2 3 4 5 6 7 8 9 (7.0, 1.3, I)	1 3 1 2 1 1 1 2 3 4 5 6 7 8 9 (5.0, 1.4, I)	(121-124)
- no response to prior SMT	1 2 3 2 1 1 2 3 4 5 6 7 8 9 (4.0, 1.0, I)	1 3 1 2 1 1 1 2 3 4 5 6 7 8 9 (3.0, 1.3, I)	1 1 1 1 4 1 1 2 3 4 5 6 7 8 9 (5.0, 1.3, I)	1 4 1 1 1 1 1 2 3 4 5 6 7 8 9 (2.0, 1.2, I)	(125-128)
- unfavorable response to prior SMT	3 2 3 1 1 2 3 4 5 6 7 8 9 (2.0, 0.9, A)	6 1 1 1 1 2 3 4 5 6 7 8 9 (1.0, 0.8, A)	3 2 1 3 1 2 3 4 5 6 7 8 9 (2.0, 1.1, I)	7 1 1 1 2 3 4 5 6 7 8 9 (1.0, 0.7, A)	(129-132)

Appropriateness scale: 1 = extremely inappropriate, 5 = uncertain, 9 = extremely appropriate.

```
Chapter 10                                NO OTHER ADEQUATE CONSERVATIVE       NONMANIPULATIVE CONSERVATIVE CARE
CERVICAL SPINAL MANIPULATION OR MOBILIZATION  CARE FOR THIS EPISODE             FOR THIS EPISODE HAS FAILED
IS INDICATED FOR CHRONIC INTERMITTENT     ------------------------------------  -----------------------------------
HEADACHE AND:                             Mobilization      Manipulation        Mobilization      Manipulation

A. Throbbing with prodrome AND

   1. Cervical signs and/or symptoms AND

      a. No clinical risk factors for
         radiographic contraindications to
         cervical manipulation, and no
         cervical radiographs
                                          1   2     6       2 1 1   2 2 1         1 2 2 2 2         2 2 1 2 2    
         - no prior SMT                   1 2 3 4 5 6 7 8 9 1 2 3 4 5 6 7 8 9 1 2 3 4 5 6 7 8 9 1 2 3 4 5 6 7 8 9   (  1-  4)
                                           (6.0, 1.2, I)     (5.0, 1.9, I)     (5.0, 1.1, I)     (5.0, 1.3, I)

         - favorable experience with          1   2 1 3 2   1   1     2 3 1 1         2 1 4 2         1 2 1 2 3  
           prior SMT                      1 2 3 4 5 6 7 8 9 1 2 3 4 5 6 7 8 9 1 2 3 4 5 6 7 8 9 1 2 3 4 5 6 7 8 9   (  5-  8)
                                           (7.0, 1.2, I)     (7.0, 1.7, I)     (7.0, 0.8, I)     (7.0, 1.2, I)

                                            2 1 2 2 2       2 1 1 1 4           1 1 3 3 1         2 1 2 2 2      
         - no response to prior SMT       1 2 3 4 5 6 7 8 9 1 2 3 4 5 6 7 8 9 1 2 3 4 5 6 7 8 9 1 2 3 4 5 6 7 8 9   (  9- 12)
                                           (4.0, 1.2, I)     (4.0, 1.4, I)     (4.0, 0.9, A)     (4.0, 1.2, I)

                                          1 3 2 3           3 2 3 1             5 2 2           1 5 2   1        
         - unfavorable response to prior SMT 1 2 3 4 5 6 7 8 9 1 2 3 4 5 6 7 8 9 1 2 3 4 5 6 7 8 9 1 2 3 4 5 6 7 8 9   ( 13- 16)
                                           (3.0, 0.9, I)     (2.0, 0.9, A)     (2.0, 0.7, A)     (2.0, 0.7, A)
      b. Cervical radiographs show no
         contraindications to cervical
         manipulation
                                            1 2   1 1 4       3   1   2 2 1       1 1   2 4 1       1     2 2 3   1
         - no prior SMT                   1 2 3 4 5 6 7 8 9 1 2 3 4 5 6 7 8 9 1 2 3 4 5 6 7 8 9 1 2 3 4 5 6 7 8 9   ( 17- 20)
                                           (6.0, 1.7, D)     (6.0, 2.0, D)     (7.0, 1.1, I)     (6.0, 1.3, I)

         - favorable experience with          1 1 1   4 1 1   1 1       4 2 1         1 2 3 2 1     1   1   2 3 2
           prior SMT                      1 2 3 4 5 6 7 8 9 1 2 3 4 5 6 7 8 9 1 2 3 4 5 6 7 8 9 1 2 3 4 5 6 7 8 9   ( 21- 24)
                                           (7.0, 1.3, I)     (7.0, 1.4, A)     (7.0, 0.9, I)     (8.0, 1.3, A)

                                            3   1 3 1 1     2 1 1 1 2 2         1 1 1 2 4       1 1 1   3 2 1    
         - no response to prior SMT       1 2 3 4 5 6 7 8 9 1 2 3 4 5 6 7 8 9 1 2 3 4 5 6 7 8 9 1 2 3 4 5 6 7 8 9   ( 25- 28)
                                           (5.0, 1.4, I)     (4.0, 1.7, I)     (5.0, 1.1, A)     (5.0, 1.4, I)

                                          3 1 1 2 2         3 2 2 1 1         1 2 1 3 2         2 3 1 2   1      
         - unfavorable response to prior SMT 1 2 3 4 5 6 7 8 9 1 2 3 4 5 6 7 8 9 1 2 3 4 5 6 7 8 9 1 2 3 4 5 6 7 8 9   ( 29- 32)
                                           (3.0, 1.4, I)     (2.0, 1.1, A)     (4.0, 1.1, I)     (2.0, 1.2, I)
```

Appropriateness scale: 1 = extremely inappropriate, 5 = uncertain, 9 = extremely appropriate.

```
Chapter 10                              NO OTHER ADEQUATE CONSERVATIVE        NONMANIPULATIVE CONSERVATIVE CARE
CERVICAL SPINAL MANIPULATION OR            CARE FOR THIS EPISODE               FOR THIS EPISODE HAS FAILED
MOBILIZATION IS INDICATED FOR          -----------------------------------  -----------------------------------
CHRONIC INTERMITTENT HEADACHE AND:      Mobilization      Manipulation       Mobilization      Manipulation

  2. No cervical signs and/or symptoms
     AND

     a. No clinical risk factors for
        radiographic contraindications to
        cervical manipulation, and no
        cervical radiographs
                                        1 2 1   5         3 1 1 3 1             2 3 1 3       2 1 2 2   2
        - no prior SMT                  1 2 3 4 5 6 7 8 9 1 2 3 4 5 6 7 8 9 1 2 3 4 5 6 7 8 9 1 2 3 4 5 6 7 8 9   ( 33- 36)
                                          (5.0, 1.3, I)     (3.0, 1.3, I)     (4.0, 1.0, A)     (3.0, 1.4, I)

        - favorable experience with     1       4 2 1   1 1   1   2 4     1       1 3 3 1   1     1 2 2 1 2   1
          prior SMT                     1 2 3 4 5 6 7 8 9 1 2 3 4 5 6 7 8 9 1 2 3 4 5 6 7 8 9 1 2 3 4 5 6 7 8 9   ( 37- 40)
                                          (5.0, 1.3, I)     (6.0, 1.4, I)     (6.0, 1.0, A)     (5.0, 1.4, I)

                                        1 1 2 4       1   1 2 2 3         1   1 1 4 2     1     3 1 2 2       1
        - no response to prior SMT      1 2 3 4 5 6 7 8 9 1 2 3 4 5 6 7 8 9 1 2 3 4 5 6 7 8 9 1 2 3 4 5 6 7 8 9   ( 41- 44)
                                          (4.0, 1.2, I)     (3.0, 1.3, I)     (4.0, 1.0, I)     (4.0, 1.6, I)

                                        3 4 1     1       4 3 1   1         2 2 4     1       2 3 2 1 1
        - unfavorable response to prior SMT
                                        1 2 3 4 5 6 7 8 9 1 2 3 4 5 6 7 8 9 1 2 3 4 5 6 7 8 9 1 2 3 4 5 6 7 8 9   ( 45- 48)
                                          (2.0, 0.9, A)     (2.0, 0.9, A)     (3.0, 1.0, A)     (2.0, 1.0, A)

     b. Cervical radiographs show no
        contraindications to cervical
        manipulation
                                        1   2   3 1 1   1 1 1   3 1 2     1       2 4   2   1   1 1   4 1   1 1
        - no prior SMT                  1 2 3 4 5 6 7 8 9 1 2 3 4 5 6 7 8 9 1 2 3 4 5 6 7 8 9 1 2 3 4 5 6 7 8 9   ( 49- 52)
                                          (5.0, 1.7, I)     (4.0, 1.7, I)     (5.0, 1.1, I)     (5.0, 1.4, I)

        - favorable experience with     1         6   1 1 1   1   1 2 3   1         3 3 1 1 1     1 1 1 2 2 1 1
          prior SMT                     1 2 3 4 5 6 7 8 9 1 2 3 4 5 6 7 8 9 1 2 3 4 5 6 7 8 9 1 2 3 4 5 6 7 8 9   ( 53- 56)
                                          (6.0, 1.1, I)     (6.0, 1.7, I)     (6.0, 1.0, I)     (6.0, 1.4, I)

                                        1   1 4 2       1 1 2 1 2 1 1     1     1 5   2     1   2 2 1 1 2     1
        - no response to prior SMT      1 2 3 4 5 6 7 8 9 1 2 3 4 5 6 7 8 9 1 2 3 4 5 6 7 8 9 1 2 3 4 5 6 7 8 9   ( 57- 60)
                                          (4.0, 1.2, I)     (4.0, 1.8, I)     (4.0, 1.1, A)     (4.0, 1.8, I)

                                        2 3 2 1     1     3 3 1 1 1         1 3 2 1 1     1   2 2 3 1 1
        - unfavorable response to prior SMT
                                        1 2 3 4 5 6 7 8 9 1 2 3 4 5 6 7 8 9 1 2 3 4 5 6 7 8 9 1 2 3 4 5 6 7 8 9   ( 61- 64)
                                          (2.0, 1.2, A)     (2.0, 1.0, A)     (3.0, 1.4, I)     (3.0, 1.0, A)
```

Appropriateness scale: 1 = extremely inappropriate, 5 = uncertain, 9 = extremely appropriate.

Chapter 10 CERVICAL SPINAL MANIPULATION OR MOBILIZATION IS INDICATED FOR CHRONIC INTERMITTENT HEADACHE AND:	NO OTHER ADEQUATE CONSERVATIVE CARE FOR THIS EPISODE		NONMANIPULATIVE CONSERVATIVE CARE FOR THIS EPISODE HAS FAILED		
	Mobilization	Manipulation	Mobilization	Manipulation	
B. Throbbing with no prodrome AND					
1. Cervical signs and/or symptoms AND					
a. No clinical risk factors for radiographic contraindications to cervical manipulation, and no cervical radiographs					
- no prior SMT	1 1 1 4 2 1 2 3 4 5 6 7 8 9 (6.0, 0.9, I)	2 1 1 1 2 2 1 2 3 4 5 6 7 8 9 (5.0, 1.7, I)	2 3 4 1 2 3 4 5 6 7 8 9 (6.0, 0.7, I)	1 1 2 2 2 1 1 2 3 4 5 6 7 8 9 (6.0, 1.3, I)	(65- 68)
- favorable experience with prior SMT	1 3 3 2 1 2 3 4 5 6 7 8 9 (7.0, 0.9, I)	1 1 5 2 1 2 3 4 5 6 7 8 9 (7.0, 0.7, A)	7 2 1 2 3 4 5 6 7 8 9 (7.0, 0.2, A)	6 2 1 1 2 3 4 5 6 7 8 9 (7.0, 0.4, A)	(69- 72)
- no response to prior SMT	3 2 3 1 1 2 3 4 5 6 7 8 9 (4.0, 0.9, I)	1 1 2 1 3 1 1 2 3 4 5 6 7 8 9 (4.0, 1.3, I)	1 3 2 2 1 1 2 3 4 5 6 7 8 9 (5.0, 1.0, A)	1 1 3 1 2 1 1 2 3 4 5 6 7 8 9 (4.0, 1.2, I)	(73- 76)
- unfavorable response to prior SMT	1 2 4 2 1 2 3 4 5 6 7 8 9 (3.0, 0.7, A)	2 3 3 1 1 2 3 4 5 6 7 8 9 (2.0, 0.8, A)	1 2 3 2 1 1 2 3 4 5 6 7 8 9 (3.0, 0.9, I)	1 3 3 1 1 1 2 3 4 5 6 7 8 9 (3.0, 0.9, A)	(77- 80)
b. Cervical radiographs show no contraindications to cervical manipulation					
- no prior SMT	2 2 3 2 1 2 3 4 5 6 7 8 9 (7.0, 1.1, I)	1 2 1 1 1 3 1 2 3 4 5 6 7 8 9 (6.0, 1.7, I)	1 1 5 2 1 2 3 4 5 6 7 8 9 (7.0, 0.6, A)	1 3 2 2 1 1 2 3 4 5 6 7 8 9 (7.0, 1.0, I)	(81- 84)
- favorable experience with prior SMT	1 1 3 3 1 1 2 3 4 5 6 7 8 9 (7.0, 1.0, A)	1 1 2 4 1 1 2 3 4 5 6 7 8 9 (8.0, 1.1, A)	5 3 1 1 2 3 4 5 6 7 8 9 (7.0, 0.6, A)	4 3 2 1 2 3 4 5 6 7 8 9 (8.0, 0.7, A)	(85- 88)
- no response to prior SMT	3 1 2 2 1 1 2 3 4 5 6 7 8 9 (5.0, 1.3, I)	1 2 1 2 2 1 1 2 3 4 5 6 7 8 9 (5.0, 1.4, I)	3 2 3 1 1 2 3 4 5 6 7 8 9 (5.0, 1.1, A)	1 1 3 2 1 1 1 2 3 4 5 6 7 8 9 (5.0, 1.2, I)	(89- 92)
- unfavorable response to prior SMT	3 2 2 2 1 2 3 4 5 6 7 8 9 (3.0, 1.0, I)	4 2 2 1 1 2 3 4 5 6 7 8 9 (3.0, 0.9, I)	1 3 3 2 1 2 3 4 5 6 7 8 9 (4.0, 0.8, I)	2 3 3 1 1 2 3 4 5 6 7 8 9 (3.0, 0.9, I)	(93- 96)

Appropriateness scale: 1 = extremely inappropriate, 5 = uncertain, 9 = extremely appropriate.

```
Chapter 10                                  NO OTHER ADEQUATE CONSERVATIVE       NONMANIPULATIVE CONSERVATIVE CARE
CERVICAL SPINAL MANIPULATION OR MOBILIZATION    CARE FOR THIS EPISODE              FOR THIS EPISODE HAS FAILED
IS INDICATED FOR CHRONIC INTERMITTENT       ----------------------------------   ----------------------------------
HEADACHE AND:                                 Mobilization      Manipulation       Mobilization      Manipulation

  2. No cervical signs and/or symptoms
     AND

     a. No clinical risk factors for
        radiographic contraindications to
        cervical manipulation, and no
        cervical radiographs
                                              3 1 5         1 2 1 4   1             1 5 2 1       2 2 1 3   1
      - no prior SMT                      1 2 3 4 5 6 7 8 9 1 2 3 4 5 6 7 8 9 1 2 3 4 5 6 7 8 9 1 2 3 4 5 6 7 8 9      ( 97-100)
                                            (5.0, 0.8, I)     (4.0, 1.1, I)     (5.0, 0.6, A)     (4.0, 1.3, I)

                                              1   2 4 1 1   1 1   1 1 4   1           2 3 3 1     1 1   2 2 3
      - favorable experience with         1 2 3 4 5 6 7 8 9 1 2 3 4 5 6 7 8 9 1 2 3 4 5 6 7 8 9 1 2 3 4 5 6 7 8 9      (101-104)
        prior SMT                           (6.0, 0.9, I)     (6.0, 1.6, I)     (6.0, 0.8, I)     (6.0, 1.3, I)

                                            3 1 4     1     2 1 3 2 1           1 1 3 3   1     1 1 2 3 1 1
      - no response to prior SMT          1 2 3 4 5 6 7 8 9 1 2 3 4 5 6 7 8 9 1 2 3 4 5 6 7 8 9 1 2 3 4 5 6 7 8 9      (105-108)
                                            (4.0, 1.1, I)     (3.0, 1.0, I)     (4.0, 1.0, I)     (4.0, 1.1, I)

                                          1 6 1 1           5 3   1             4 3 1 1         2 4 2   1
      - unfavorable response to prior SMT 1 2 3 4 5 6 7 8 9 1 2 3 4 5 6 7 8 9 1 2 3 4 5 6 7 8 9 1 2 3 4 5 6 7 8 9      (109-112)
                                            (2.0, 0.4, A)     (1.0, 0.7, A)     (3.0, 0.8, A)     (2.0, 0.8, A)
     b. Cervical radiographs show no
        contraindications to cervical
        manipulation
                                              2 1 3 1 2     1 1   3 1 2 1           2 4   3         1 2 4 1   1
      - no prior SMT                      1 2 3 4 5 6 7 8 9 1 2 3 4 5 6 7 8 9 1 2 3 4 5 6 7 8 9 1 2 3 4 5 6 7 8 9      (113-116)
                                            (5.0, 1.1, I)     (4.0, 1.4, I)     (5.0, 0.9, I)     (5.0, 0.9, A)

                                                1   5 1 2       1     3 4 1           1 3 4 1           3 2 3 1
      - favorable experience with         1 2 3 4 5 6 7 8 9 1 2 3 4 5 6 7 8 9 1 2 3 4 5 6 7 8 9 1 2 3 4 5 6 7 8 9      (117-120)
        prior SMT                           (6.0, 0.8, I)     (7.0, 0.9, I)     (7.0, 0.7, I)     (6.0, 0.9, I)

                                          1   1 4 2   1     1 1 2 2 1 2           1 4 1 2 1       1 2 2 2 2
      - no response to prior SMT          1 2 3 4 5 6 7 8 9 1 2 3 4 5 6 7 8 9 1 2 3 4 5 6 7 8 9 1 2 3 4 5 6 7 8 9      (121-124)
                                            (4.0, 1.0, I)     (4.0, 1.3, I)     (4.0, 1.0, A)     (4.0, 1.1, I)

                                          2 3 3 1           2 4 1 1 1         1 3 3   2         1 5 2   1
      - unfavorable response to prior SMT 1 2 3 4 5 6 7 8 9 1 2 3 4 5 6 7 8 9 1 2 3 4 5 6 7 8 9 1 2 3 4 5 6 7 8 9      (125-128)
                                            (2.0, 0.8, A)     (2.0, 0.9, A)     (3.0, 1.0, A)     (2.0, 0.7, A)
```

Appropriateness scale: 1 = extremely inappropriate, 5 = uncertain, 9 = extremely appropriate.

```
Chapter 10                                      NO OTHER ADEQUATE CONSERVATIVE         NONMANIPULATIVE CONSERVATIVE CARE
CERVICAL SPINAL MANIPULATION OR MOBILIZATION         CARE FOR THIS EPISODE                FOR THIS EPISODE HAS FAILED
IS INDICATED FOR CHRONIC INTERMITTENT          -------------------------------------   ---------------------------------
HEADACHE AND:                                     Mobilization       Manipulation        Mobilization       Manipulation

C. Non-throbbing with prodrome AND

   1. Cervical signs and/or symptoms AND

      a. No clinical risk factors for
         radiographic contraindications to
         cervical manipulation, and no
         cervical radiographs
                                                   1 1 2 4 1       1   1 2 2 2 1           3 2 4           1 3 3 1 1
         - no prior SMT                          1 2 3 4 5 6 7 8 9 1 2 3 4 5 6 7 8 9 1 2 3 4 5 6 7 8 9 1 2 3 4 5 6 7 8 9   (129-132)
                                                   (6.0, 0.9, A)     (5.0, 1.3, I)     (6.0, 0.8, I)     (6.0, 0.9, A)

         - favorable experience with               1       3 3 1 1 1   1   1 1 3 1 1           2 4 2 1         1 2 3 2 1
           prior SMT                             1 2 3 4 5 6 7 8 9 1 2 3 4 5 6 7 8 9 1 2 3 4 5 6 7 8 9 1 2 3 4 5 6 7 8 9   (133-136)
                                                   (7.0, 1.1, I)     (7.0, 1.8, I)     (7.0, 0.7, A)     (7.0, 0.9, I)

                                                   1   3 4     1   1 1 2   3 1   1         3 3 2     1     1 1 2 2 1 1   1
         - no response to prior SMT              1 2 3 4 5 6 7 8 9 1 2 3 4 5 6 7 8 9 1 2 3 4 5 6 7 8 9 1 2 3 4 5 6 7 8 9   (137-140)
                                                   (5.0, 1.0, A)     (5.0, 1.7, I)     (5.0, 1.0, A)     (5.0, 1.6, I)

                                                 1 2 3 2 1         3 1 3   2         1 1 3 2 2         1 2 4   1 1
         - unfavorable response to prior SMT     1 2 3 4 5 6 7 8 9 1 2 3 4 5 6 7 8 9 1 2 3 4 5 6 7 8 9 1 2 3 4 5 6 7 8 9   (141-144)
                                                   (3.0, 0.9, I)     (3.0, 1.2, A)     (3.0, 1.0, I)     (3.0, 1.0, A)
      b. Cervical radiographs show no
         contraindications to cervical
         manipulation
                                                       1 1 3 3   1       3   3 1 1 1           2 6   1         1 4 2   2
         - no prior SMT                          1 2 3 4 5 6 7 8 9 1 2 3 4 5 6 7 8 9 1 2 3 4 5 6 7 8 9 1 2 3 4 5 6 7 8 9   (145-148)
                                                   (6.0, 1.0, I)     (6.0, 1.3, I)     (7.0, 0.4, A)     (6.0, 1.0, I)

         - favorable experience with                   1     6 1 1     1   1   4 2 1             5 3 1             4 3 2
           prior SMT                             1 2 3 4 5 6 7 8 9 1 2 3 4 5 6 7 8 9 1 2 3 4 5 6 7 8 9 1 2 3 4 5 6 7 8 9   (149-152)
                                                   (7.0, 0.7, A)     (7.0, 1.1, A)     (7.0, 0.6, A)     (8.0, 0.7, A)

                                                     1 2 3 2   1   1 1 1 1 2 1 1 1           2 3 3   1       1   1 3 2 1 1
         - no response to prior SMT              1 2 3 4 5 6 7 8 9 1 2 3 4 5 6 7 8 9 1 2 3 4 5 6 7 8 9 1 2 3 4 5 6 7 8 9   (153-156)
                                                   (5.0, 1.0, A)     (5.0, 1.8, I)     (5.0, 0.9, A)     (5.0, 1.2, I)

                                                   1 4 1 3         2 2 2 1 1 1         1 3 2 3             2 3 2 1 1
         - unfavorable response to prior SMT     1 2 3 4 5 6 7 8 9 1 2 3 4 5 6 7 8 9 1 2 3 4 5 6 7 8 9 1 2 3 4 5 6 7 8 9   (157-160)
                                                   (3.0, 0.9, I)     (3.0, 1.3, I)     (4.0, 0.9, I)     (3.0, 1.0, I)
```

Appropriateness scale: 1 = extremely inappropriate, 5 = uncertain, 9 = extremely appropriate.

Chapter 10 CERVICAL SPINAL MANIPULATION OR MOBILIZATION IS INDICATED FOR CHRONIC INTERMITTENT HEADACHE AND:	NO OTHER ADEQUATE CONSERVATIVE CARE FOR THIS EPISODE Mobilization	 Manipulation	NONMANIPULATIVE CONSERVATIVE CARE FOR THIS EPISODE HAS FAILED Mobilization	 Manipulation	
2. No cervical signs and/or symptoms AND					
a. No clinical risk factors for radiographic contraindications to cervical manipulation, and no cervical radiographs					
- no prior SMT	1 _ 3 1 3 _ 1 _ _ 1 2 3 4 5 6 7 8 9 (4.0, 1.3, I)	1 1 2 3 _ 1 1 _ _ 1 2 3 4 5 6 7 8 9 (4.0, 1.3, I)	_ _ 1 1 4 2 1 _ _ 1 2 3 4 5 6 7 8 9 (5.0, 0.8, A)	_ 1 2 1 2 1 2 _ _ 1 2 3 4 5 6 7 8 9 (5.0, 1.4, I)	(161-164)
- favorable experience with prior SMT	1 _ _ 1 2 2 2 1 _ 1 2 3 4 5 6 7 8 9 (6.0, 1.4, I)	1 _ _ 1 1 5 _ 1 _ 1 2 3 4 5 6 7 8 9 (6.0, 1.1, A)	_ _ _ 1 2 3 2 1 _ 1 2 3 4 5 6 7 8 9 (6.0, 0.9, I)	_ _ 1 1 2 _ 4 1 _ 1 2 3 4 5 6 7 8 9 (7.0, 1.3, I)	(165-168)
- no response to prior SMT	1 1 3 3 _ 1 _ _ _ 1 2 3 4 5 6 7 8 9 (3.0, 1.1, I)	2 1 3 1 1 _ 1 _ _ 1 2 3 4 5 6 7 8 9 (3.0, 1.3, I)	_ _ 2 3 3 _ 1 _ _ 1 2 3 4 5 6 7 8 9 (4.0, 0.9, I)	1 _ 3 2 2 _ 1 _ _ 1 2 3 4 5 6 7 8 9 (4.0, 1.2, I)	(169-172)
- unfavorable response to prior SMT	3 4 1 _ 1 _ _ _ _ 1 2 3 4 5 6 7 8 9 (2.0, 0.8, A)	4 3 _ 1 1 _ _ _ _ 1 2 3 4 5 6 7 8 9 (2.0, 1.0, A)	1 2 3 2 1 _ _ _ _ 1 2 3 4 5 6 7 8 9 (3.0, 0.9, I)	2 3 2 1 1 _ _ _ _ 1 2 3 4 5 6 7 8 9 (2.0, 1.0, A)	(173-176)
b. Cervical radiographs show no contraindications to cervical manipulation					
- no prior SMT	_ _ 2 1 3 1 2 _ _ 1 2 3 4 5 6 7 8 9 (5.0, 1.1, I)	1 _ _ 4 1 1 2 _ _ 1 2 3 4 5 6 7 8 9 (4.0, 1.3, I)	_ _ _ 2 4 _ 3 _ _ 1 2 3 4 5 6 7 8 9 (5.0, 0.9, I)	_ _ _ 2 4 1 1 1 _ 1 2 3 4 5 6 7 8 9 (5.0, 0.9, A)	(177-180)
- favorable experience with prior SMT	_ _ 1 _ 1 4 _ 3 _ 1 2 3 4 5 6 7 8 9 (6.0, 1.1, I)	1 _ _ _ 1 2 4 1 _ 1 2 3 4 5 6 7 8 9 (7.0, 1.2, I)	_ _ _ _ 1 2 3 2 1 1 2 3 4 5 6 7 8 9 (7.0, 0.9, I)	_ _ _ _ 2 1 4 1 1 1 2 3 4 5 6 7 8 9 (7.0, 0.9, I)	(181-184)
- no response to prior SMT	1 1 _ 4 2 _ 1 _ _ 1 2 3 4 5 6 7 8 9 (4.0, 1.1, I)	1 2 1 2 1 1 1 _ _ 1 2 3 4 5 6 7 8 9 (4.0, 1.6, I)	_ _ 1 4 1 2 1 _ _ 1 2 3 4 5 6 7 8 9 (4.0, 1.0, A)	_ 1 2 3 _ 1 2 _ _ 1 2 3 4 5 6 7 8 9 (4.0, 1.3, I)	(185-188)
- unfavorable response to prior SMT	3 2 2 1 1 _ _ _ _ 1 2 3 4 5 6 7 8 9 (2.0, 1.1, A)	3 3 1 _ 2 _ _ _ _ 1 2 3 4 5 6 7 8 9 (2.0, 1.1, A)	1 3 3 _ 2 _ _ _ _ 1 2 3 4 5 6 7 8 9 (3.0, 1.0, A)	1 4 2 _ 1 1 _ _ _ 1 2 3 4 5 6 7 8 9 (2.0, 1.1, A)	(189-192)

Appropriateness scale: 1 = extremely inappropriate, 5 = uncertain, 9 = extremely appropriate.

```
Chapter 10                                NO OTHER ADEQUATE CONSERVATIVE       NONMANIPULATIVE CONSERVATIVE CARE
CERVICAL SPINAL MANIPULATION OR MOBILIZATION   CARE FOR THIS EPISODE            FOR THIS EPISODE HAS FAILED
IS INDICATED FOR CHRONIC INTERMITTENT     -----------------------------------  ----------------------------------
HEADACHE AND:                               Mobilization      Manipulation      Mobilization      Manipulation

D. Non-throbbing with no prodrome AND

  1. Cervical signs and/or symptoms AND

    a. No clinical risk factors for
       radiographic contraindications to
       cervical manipulation, and no
       cervical radiographs
                                              1 1 4 3    2       2   4 1            4 3 2      1 1 1 1 1 4
       - no prior SMT                   1 2 3 4 5 6 7 8 9 1 2 3 4 5 6 7 8 9 1 2 3 4 5 6 7 8 9 1 2 3 4 5 6 7 8 9     (193-196)
                                          (6.0, 0.7, I)    (7.0, 1.9, I)     (7.0, 0.7, I)     (7.0, 1.6, I)

       - favorable experience with            1   1 2 5  1 1       1 1 5              5 2 2   1         2 5 1
         prior SMT                      1 2 3 4 5 6 7 8 9 1 2 3 4 5 6 7 8 9 1 2 3 4 5 6 7 8 9 1 2 3 4 5 6 7 8 9     (197-200)
                                          (8.0, 0.9, A)    (8.0, 1.8, I)     (7.0, 0.7, A)     (8.0, 1.0, A)

                                            2 1 3 2   1  2     2 1 3 1        1   3 3 1   1 1 1   2   2 2   1
       - no response to prior SMT       1 2 3 4 5 6 7 8 9 1 2 3 4 5 6 7 8 9 1 2 3 4 5 6 7 8 9 1 2 3 4 5 6 7 8 9     (201-204)
                                          (5.0, 1.1, I)    (5.0, 1.7, I)     (6.0, 1.1, I)     (6.0, 2.0, I)

                                        1 2 1 2 3         2 1 2 1 2 1       1 1 2 1 4         1 2 2 1 2 1
       - unfavorable response to prior SMT 1 2 3 4 5 6 7 8 9 1 2 3 4 5 6 7 8 9 1 2 3 4 5 6 7 8 9 1 2 3 4 5 6 7 8 9  (205-208)
                                          (4.0, 1.2, I)    (3.0, 1.4, I)     (4.0, 1.2, I)     (3.0, 1.3, I)
    b. Cervical radiographs show no
       contraindications to cervical
       manipulation
                                                1 3 2 1 2       1 1 2 1 1 3             6 1 2           2 2 2 3
       - no prior SMT                   1 2 3 4 5 6 7 8 9 1 2 3 4 5 6 7 8 9 1 2 3 4 5 6 7 8 9 1 2 3 4 5 6 7 8 9     (209-212)
                                          (7.0, 1.1, I)    (7.0, 1.6, I)     (7.0, 0.6, A)     (8.0, 1.0, A)

       - favorable experience with              1   3 2 3       1   1 2 1 4             3 2 4           1 2 2 4
         prior SMT                      1 2 3 4 5 6 7 8 9 1 2 3 4 5 6 7 8 9 1 2 3 4 5 6 7 8 9 1 2 3 4 5 6 7 8 9     (213-216)
                                          (8.0, 1.0, A)    (8.0, 1.3, A)     (8.0, 0.8, A)     (8.0, 0.9, A)

                                            2   3 1 1 2  1 1     3   2 2        1   3 2 2   1   1   1 2 1 2 1 1
       - no response to prior SMT       1 2 3 4 5 6 7 8 9 1 2 3 4 5 6 7 8 9 1 2 3 4 5 6 7 8 9 1 2 3 4 5 6 7 8 9     (217-220)
                                          (5.0, 1.4, I)    (5.0, 1.9, I)     (6.0, 1.2, I)     (6.0, 1.7, I)

                                          2 2 1 2 2       2 1 1 1 3   1       2 1 2 3 1       1 2 1 1 3   1
       - unfavorable response to prior SMT 1 2 3 4 5 6 7 8 9 1 2 3 4 5 6 7 8 9 1 2 3 4 5 6 7 8 9 1 2 3 4 5 6 7 8 9  (221-224)
                                          (4.0, 1.3, I)    (4.0, 1.7, I)     (4.0, 1.1, I)     (4.0, 1.6, I)
```

Appropriateness scale: 1 = extremely inappropriate, 5 = uncertain, 9 = extremely appropriate.

Chapter 10 CERVICAL SPINAL MANIPULATION OR MOBILIZATION IS INDICATED FOR CHRONIC INTERMITTENT HEADACHE AND:	NO OTHER ADEQUATE CONSERVATIVE CARE FOR THIS EPISODE Mobilization	 Manipulation	NONMANIPULATIVE CONSERVATIVE CARE FOR THIS EPISODE HAS FAILED Mobilization	 Manipulation	
2. No cervical signs and/or symptoms AND					
a. No clinical risk factors for radiographic contraindications to cervical manipulation, and no cervical radiographs					
- no prior SMT	1 1 3 2 1 1 1 2 3 4 5 6 7 8 9 (4.0, 1.1, I)	2 2 2 1 2 1 2 3 4 5 6 7 8 9 (4.0, 1.7, I)	1 4 2 2 1 2 3 4 5 6 7 8 9 (5.0, 0.8, A)	1 1 1 1 2 1 2 1 2 3 4 5 6 7 8 9 (5.0, 2.0, D)	(225-228)
- favorable experience with prior SMT	1 3 2 1 2 1 2 3 4 5 6 7 8 9 (6.0, 1.1, I)	1 1 1 2 1 2 1 1 2 3 4 5 6 7 8 9 (5.0, 1.6, I)	1 4 2 1 1 1 2 3 4 5 6 7 8 9 (6.0, 0.9, I)	2 1 2 4 1 2 3 4 5 6 7 8 9 (6.0, 1.7, I)	(229-232)
- no response to prior SMT	1 3 1 2 2 1 2 3 4 5 6 7 8 9 (4.0, 1.2, I)	3 1 2 1 2 1 2 3 4 5 6 7 8 9 (4.0, 1.3, I)	2 3 1 3 1 2 3 4 5 6 7 8 9 (4.0, 1.0, A)	1 2 3 2 1 1 2 3 4 5 6 7 8 9 (4.0, 1.2, I)	(233-236)
- unfavorable response to prior SMT	2 3 2 1 1 1 2 3 4 5 6 7 8 9 (2.0, 1.0, A)	3 3 1 2 1 2 3 4 5 6 7 8 9 (2.0, 1.1, A)	1 2 4 1 1 1 2 3 4 5 6 7 8 9 (3.0, 0.8, A)	1 4 2 1 1 1 2 3 4 5 6 7 8 9 (2.0, 1.1, A)	(237-240)
b. Cervical radiographs show no contraindications to cervical manipulation					
- no prior SMT	1 1 4 3 1 2 3 4 5 6 7 8 9 (5.0, 1.0, I)	1 1 2 3 1 1 1 2 3 4 5 6 7 8 9 (5.0, 1.4, I)	5 1 3 1 2 3 4 5 6 7 8 9 (5.0, 0.8, I)	1 2 3 1 1 1 1 2 3 4 5 6 7 8 9 (5.0, 1.4, I)	(241-244)
- favorable experience with prior SMT	1 1 3 1 3 1 2 3 4 5 6 7 8 9 (6.0, 1.2, I)	1 1 4 3 1 2 3 4 5 6 7 8 9 (6.0, 1.3, I)	4 2 2 1 1 2 3 4 5 6 7 8 9 (7.0, 0.9, I)	4 1 3 1 1 2 3 4 5 6 7 8 9 (7.0, 1.0, I)	(245-248)
- no response to prior SMT	2 2 2 3 1 2 3 4 5 6 7 8 9 (5.0, 1.0, A)	1 4 2 2 1 2 3 4 5 6 7 8 9 (3.0, 1.3, I)	4 2 3 1 2 3 4 5 6 7 8 9 (5.0, 0.8, A)	3 3 2 1 1 2 3 4 5 6 7 8 9 (4.0, 1.2, I)	(249-252)
- unfavorable response to prior SMT	1 3 3 2 1 2 3 4 5 6 7 8 9 (3.0, 1.0, A)	2 3 2 2 1 2 3 4 5 6 7 8 9 (2.0, 1.1, A)	1 6 2 1 2 3 4 5 6 7 8 9 (3.0, 0.6, A)	5 2 1 1 1 2 3 4 5 6 7 8 9 (2.0, 1.1, A)	(253-256)

Appropriateness scale: 1 = extremely inappropriate, 5 = uncertain, 9 = extremely appropriate.

Chapter 11 CERVICAL SPINAL MANIPULATION OR MOBILIZATION IS APPROPRIATE WITH:	NO OTHER ADEQUATE CONSERVATIVE CARE FOR THIS EPISODE		NONMANIPULATIVE CONSERVATIVE CARE FOR THIS EPISODE HAS FAILED		
	Mobilization	Manipulation	Mobilization	Manipulation	
A. Persistent neuralgic pain consistent with a cranial nerve distribution	6 3 1 2 3 4 5 6 7 8 9 (2.0, 0.3, A)	6 2 1 1 2 3 4 5 6 7 8 9 (2.0, 0.4, A)	3 4 2 1 2 3 4 5 6 7 8 9 (3.0, 0.6, A)	2 5 1 1 1 2 3 4 5 6 7 8 9 (3.0, 0.7, A)	(1- 4)
B. Insidious facial palsy (including Bell's palsy)	4 3 1 1 1 2 3 4 5 6 7 8 9 (2.0, 0.9, A)	5 1 1 1 1 1 2 3 4 5 6 7 8 9 (1.0, 1.1, A)	4 2 1 1 1 1 2 3 4 5 6 7 8 9 (2.0, 1.1, A)	5 2 1 1 1 2 3 4 5 6 7 8 9 (1.0, 1.6, A)	(5- 8)
C. Idiopathic insidious vertigo and/or dizziness	5 1 3 1 2 3 4 5 6 7 8 9 (2.0, 0.8, I)	1 1 4 2 1 1 2 3 4 5 6 7 8 9 (3.0, 1.0, I)	1 3 3 2 1 2 3 4 5 6 7 8 9 (4.0, 1.0, I)	2 2 3 1 1 1 2 3 4 5 6 7 8 9 (4.0, 1.3, I)	(9- 12)
D. Spasmodic torticollis in the absence of congenital, postsurgical or post-fracture etiologies	2 1 2 4 1 2 3 4 5 6 7 8 9 (3.0, 1.4, I)	4 1 1 2 1 1 2 3 4 5 6 7 8 9 (2.0, 1.6, I)	1 2 1 4 1 1 2 3 4 5 6 7 8 9 (5.0, 1.6, I)	2 3 2 1 1 1 2 3 4 5 6 7 8 9 (2.0, 1.7, I)	(13- 16)
E. Idiopathic insidious pharyngeal dysfunction	2 6 1 1 2 3 4 5 6 7 8 9 (2.0, 0.3, A)	3 3 2 1 1 2 3 4 5 6 7 8 9 (2.0, 0.8, A)	1 3 2 1 2 1 2 3 4 5 6 7 8 9 (3.0, 1.1, I)	2 1 5 1 1 2 3 4 5 6 7 8 9 (3.0, 0.8, A)	(17- 20)

Appropriateness scale: 1 = extremely inappropriate, 5 = uncertain, 9 = extremely appropriate.

```
Chapter 12
CERVICAL SPINAL MANIPULATION OR MOBILIZATION          Manipulation         Manipulation
IS APPROPRIATE WITH:                                    excluding            including
AN OTHERWISE APPROPRIATE INDICATION FOR                 rotation             rotation
CERVICAL SPINE MANIPULATIVE THERAPY AND  Mobilization   -extension          -extension

A. Radiographic evidence of mild to moderate
   generalized diffuse demineralization of      1 2 1 5              1 2 3 2 1        1 1 3 2 2
   bone in the cervical spine             1 2 3 4 5 6 7 8 9  1 2 3 4 5 6 7 8 9  1 2 3 4 5 6 7 8 9   (  1-  3)
                                            (7.0, 0.9, I)      (6.0, 0.9, I)      (4.0, 1.0, A)
B. Radiographic evidence of moderate to
   severe generalized diffuse
   demineralization of bone in the cervical   1 1 3     4          3 1 4 1        6   2 1
   spine                                  1 2 3 4 5 6 7 8 9  1 2 3 4 5 6 7 8 9  1 2 3 4 5 6 7 8 9   (  4-  6)
                                            (5.0, 1.2, I)      (5.0, 0.9, I)      (1.0, 0.8, A)
C. Radiographic evidence consistent with
   possible infection or malignant neoplasm 9                  9                  9
   in the cervical spine                  1 2 3 4 5 6 7 8 9  1 2 3 4 5 6 7 8 9  1 2 3 4 5 6 7 8 9   (  7-  9)
                                            (1.0, 0.0, A)      (1.0, 0.0, A)      (1.0, 0.0, A)

D. Radiographic evidence consistent with    1 1 3 4          2 2 1 1 3          4 2 3
   Paget's disease of bone                1 2 3 4 5 6 7 8 9  1 2 3 4 5 6 7 8 9  1 2 3 4 5 6 7 8 9   ( 10- 12)
                                            (4.0, 0.8, A)      (3.0, 1.4, I)      (2.0, 0.8, A)
E. Radiographic evidence of benign bone tumor
   that has no characteristics of mechanical
   instability of the osseous structure in          3 4 1 1        1 2 3 1 1 1    2 1 3 1 1 1
   the cervical spine                     1 2 3 4 5 6 7 8 9  1 2 3 4 5 6 7 8 9  1 2 3 4 5 6 7 8 9   ( 13- 15)
                                            (6.0, 0.7, A)      (5.0, 1.1, I)      (3.0, 1.2, I)
F. Radiographic evidence of benign bone tumor
   that has characteristics of mechanical
   instability of the osseous structure in 3 5 1              8 1                9
   the cervical spine                     1 2 3 4 5 6 7 8 9  1 2 3 4 5 6 7 8 9  1 2 3 4 5 6 7 8 9   ( 16- 18)
                                            (2.0, 0.4, A)      (1.0, 0.1, A)      (1.0, 0.0, A)
G. Radiographic indications of acute
   fracture/dislocation, or
   fracture/dislocation with radiographic
   signs of ligamentous rupture or        9                  9                  9
   instability                            1 2 3 4 5 6 7 8 9  1 2 3 4 5 6 7 8 9  1 2 3 4 5 6 7 8 9   ( 19- 21)
                                            (1.0, 0.0, A)      (1.0, 0.0, A)      (1.0, 0.0, A)
H. Radiographic evidence of os odontoideum
   of:
                                          9                  9                  9
   1. Unstable nature                     1 2 3 4 5 6 7 8 9  1 2 3 4 5 6 7 8 9  1 2 3 4 5 6 7 8 9   ( 22- 24)
                                            (1.0, 0.0, A)      (1.0, 0.0, A)      (1.0, 0.0, A)

                                          2 1 3 1 2          3   4   2          5 2 2
   2. Stable nature                       1 2 3 4 5 6 7 8 9  1 2 3 4 5 6 7 8 9  1 2 3 4 5 6 7 8 9   ( 25- 27)
                                            (3.0, 1.1, I)      (3.0, 1.1, A)      (1.0, 0.7, A)
```

Appropriateness scale: 1 = extremely inappropriate, 5 = uncertain, 9 = extremely appropriate.

Chapter 12 CERVICAL SPINAL MANIPULATION OR MOBILIZATION IS APPROPRIATE WITH: AN OTHERWISE APPROPRIATE INDICATION FOR CERVICAL SPINE MANIPULATIVE THERAPY AND	Mobilization	Manipulation excluding rotation -extension	Manipulation including rotation -extension	
I. Clinical evidence of articular hypermobility				
1. No cervical spine radiographs	1 2 1 5 1 2 3 4 5 6 7 8 9 (5.0, 0.9, I)	1 2 3 2 1 1 2 3 4 5 6 7 8 9 (3.0, 0.9, I)	4 4 1 1 2 3 4 5 6 7 8 9 (2.0, 0.6, A)	(28- 30)
2. Radiographic evidence of articular hypermobility	1 2 4 2 1 2 3 4 5 6 7 8 9 (4.0, 0.7, I)	2 5 1 1 1 2 3 4 5 6 7 8 9 (2.0, 0.7, A)	6 2 1 1 2 3 4 5 6 7 8 9 (1.0, 0.4, A)	(31- 33)
J. Postsurgical joints or segments with no evidence of instability and adequate healing time AND				
1. Favorable prior response to cervical SMT since surgery	4 5 1 2 3 4 5 6 7 8 9 (7.0, 0.4, I)	1 4 3 1 1 2 3 4 5 6 7 8 9 (6.0, 0.7, I)	1 3 2 2 1 1 2 3 4 5 6 7 8 9 (5.0, 1.2, A)	(34- 36)
2. No prior response to cervical SMT since surgery	1 5 2 1 1 2 3 4 5 6 7 8 9 (5.0, 0.6, A)	1 2 3 2 1 1 2 3 4 5 6 7 8 9 (5.0, 0.9, A)	2 1 4 1 1 1 2 3 4 5 6 7 8 9 (3.0, 0.9, A)	(37- 39)
3. Unfavorable prior response to cervical SMT since surgery	3 5 1 1 2 3 4 5 6 7 8 9 (5.0, 0.4, A)	1 4 1 1 2 1 2 3 4 5 6 7 8 9 (3.0, 1.1, I)	3 2 2 2 1 2 3 4 5 6 7 8 9 (2.0, 1.2, A)	(40- 42)
K. Radiographic and clinical manifestations of non-specific and/or rheumatoid arthropathies without any radiographic evidence of cervical spine instability, anatomic subluxation or dislocation AND				
1. Characterized by episodes of acute inflammation and signs of ligamentous laxity	1 3 4 1 1 2 3 4 5 6 7 8 9 (5.0, 1.2, I)	3 1 2 1 1 1 1 2 3 4 5 6 7 8 9 (3.0, 1.8, I)	6 2 1 1 2 3 4 5 6 7 8 9 (1.0, 0.6, A)	(43- 45)
2. Characterized by subacute or chronic presentations with no signs of ligamentous laxity, ankylosis, and/or anatomic subluxation	2 4 2 1 1 2 3 4 5 6 7 8 9 (5.0, 0.8, A)	1 1 1 1 3 1 1 1 2 3 4 5 6 7 8 9 (5.0, 1.7, I)	4 1 2 1 1 1 2 3 4 5 6 7 8 9 (2.0, 1.3, A)	(46- 48)
L. Major neurologic findings	8 1 1 2 3 4 5 6 7 8 9 (1.0, 0.1, A)	9 1 2 3 4 5 6 7 8 9 (1.0, 0.0, A)	9 1 2 3 4 5 6 7 8 9 (1.0, 0.0, A)	(49- 51)
M. Connective tissue disorder				
1. Without special cervical spine radiographic studies	2 1 3 1 2 1 2 3 4 5 6 7 8 9 (3.0, 1.1, I)	4 3 2 1 2 3 4 5 6 7 8 9 (2.0, 0.7, A)	6 1 2 1 2 3 4 5 6 7 8 9 (1.0, 0.6, A)	(52- 54)
2. With special cervical spine radiographic studies	1 6 1 1 1 2 3 4 5 6 7 8 9 (5.0, 0.7, A)	1 2 1 2 2 1 1 2 3 4 5 6 7 8 9 (4.0, 1.4, I)	3 2 1 1 1 1 1 2 3 4 5 6 7 8 9 (2.0, 1.6, I)	(55- 57)

Appropriateness scale: 1 = extremely inappropriate, 5 = uncertain, 9 = extremely appropriate.

```
Chapter 13
CERVICAL SPINAL MANIPULATION OR MOBILIZATION                        Manipulation      Manipulation
IS APPROPRIATE WITH:                                                  excluding         including
AN OTHERWISE APPROPRIATE INDICATION FOR                               rotation          rotation
CERVICAL SPINE MANIPULATIVE THERAPY AND           Mobilization       -extension        -extension

A. Possible clotting disorders and/or history
   of current anti-coagulant therapy AND
                                                    1 6   1   1       3 3 2   1         4 2 3
   1. Without clotting or bleeding tests          1 2 3 4 5 6 7 8 9 1 2 3 4 5 6 7 8 9 1 2 3 4 5 6 7 8 9     ( 1-  3)
                                                    (3.0, 0.8, A)     (2.0, 0.9, A)     (2.0, 0.8, A)

   2. With abnormal clotting or bleeding          1 1 7             7   2             8   1
      tests                                       1 2 3 4 5 6 7 8 9 1 2 3 4 5 6 7 8 9 1 2 3 4 5 6 7 8 9     ( 4-  6)
                                                    (3.0, 0.3, A)     (1.0, 0.4, A)     (1.0, 0.2, A)

                                                    1   1 5   1 1       1 3 1 1 1 1 1   3 2 1 1 1     1
   3. With normal clotting or bleeding tests      1 2 3 4 5 6 7 8 9 1 2 3 4 5 6 7 8 9 1 2 3 4 5 6 7 8 9     ( 7-  9)
                                                    (5.0, 1.0, I)     (4.0, 1.7, I)     (2.0, 1.7, I)

B. Radiographic evidence of vertebral or          1   2 2 2 1   1   2 2 2   1 1   1   8         1
   carotid artery calcification                   1 2 3 4 5 6 7 8 9 1 2 3 4 5 6 7 8 9 1 2 3 4 5 6 7 8 9     ( 10- 12)
                                                    (4.0, 1.4, I)     (3.0, 1.8, I)     (1.0, 0.6, A)

C. Clinical or physical examination evidence      1   2   1 3 1 1   2 1   2 2   2     6 2       1
   of occlusive vascular disease                  1 2 3 4 5 6 7 8 9 1 2 3 4 5 6 7 8 9 1 2 3 4 5 6 7 8 9     ( 13- 15)
                                                    (6.0, 1.7, I)     (4.0, 1.8, I)     (1.0, 0.8, A)

D. Poorly controlled hypertension                   1   1 4 2 1     1 1 1   2 2 2     3 2 2 2
   (BP > 180/110)                                 1 2 3 4 5 6 7 8 9 1 2 3 4 5 6 7 8 9 1 2 3 4 5 6 7 8 9     ( 16- 18)
                                                    (5.0, 0.9, A)     (5.0, 1.7, I)     (2.0, 1.0, A)

                                                      1   2 2 2 2   1   1   1   4 2   2 1 2 1 2   1
E. Hypertension with BP < 180/110                 1 2 3 4 5 6 7 8 9 1 2 3 4 5 6 7 8 9 1 2 3 4 5 6 7 8 9     ( 19- 21)
                                                    (6.0, 1.2, I)     (7.0, 1.6, I)     (3.0, 1.6, I)
F. History of transient ischemic attack
                                                        3 5   1     1   3 2 2   1     4   3 1   1
   1. Carotid origin                              1 2 3 4 5 6 7 8 9 1 2 3 4 5 6 7 8 9 1 2 3 4 5 6 7 8 9     ( 22- 24)
                                                    (5.0, 0.6, A)     (4.0, 1.2, I)     (3.0, 1.3, A)

                                                  3 4 2             6 1 2             9
   2. Presumed vertebrobasiler                    1 2 3 4 5 6 7 8 9 1 2 3 4 5 6 7 8 9 1 2 3 4 5 6 7 8 9     ( 25- 27)
                                                    (2.0, 0.6, A)     (1.0, 0.6, A)     (1.0, 0.0, A)
G. History of cerebrovascular accident
                                                    1 3   4   1     1 2 3 2     1     6 1 1     1
   1. Carotid origin                              1 2 3 4 5 6 7 8 9 1 2 3 4 5 6 7 8 9 1 2 3 4 5 6 7 8 9     ( 28- 30)
                                                    (5.0, 1.2, I)     (3.0, 1.1, I)     (1.0, 0.9, A)

                                                  6 2 1             7 1 1             9
   2. Presumed vertebrobasiler                    1 2 3 4 5 6 7 8 9 1 2 3 4 5 6 7 8 9 1 2 3 4 5 6 7 8 9     ( 31- 33)
                                                    (1.0, 0.4, A)     (1.0, 0.3, A)     (1.0, 0.0, A)

                                                          2   4 3           2 1 3 3   1   1 2 2 1 1 1
H. Age > 65                                       1 2 3 4 5 6 7 8 9 1 2 3 4 5 6 7 8 9 1 2 3 4 5 6 7 8 9     ( 34- 36)
                                                    (7.0, 0.8, A)     (7.0, 0.9, I)     (5.0, 1.6, I)

I. History of sudden onset focal neurologic       8   1             8   1             9
   findings after cervical manipulation           1 2 3 4 5 6 7 8 9 1 2 3 4 5 6 7 8 9 1 2 3 4 5 6 7 8 9     ( 37- 39)
                                                    (1.0, 0.2, A)     (1.0, 0.2, A)     (1.0, 0.0, A)
```

Appropriateness scale: 1 = extremely inappropriate, 5 = uncertain, 9 = extremely appropriate.

Chapter 13 CERVICAL SPINAL MANIPULATION OR MOBILIZATION IS APPROPRIATE WITH: AN OTHERWISE APPROPRIATE INDICATION FOR CERVICAL SPINE MANIPULATIVE THERAPY AND	Mobilization	Manipulation excluding rotation -extension	Manipulation including rotation -extension	
J. Sustained nystagmus or dizziness during or immediately after provocative testing	7 1 1 1 2 3 4 5 6 7 8 9 (1.0, 0.3, A)	7 1 1 1 2 3 4 5 6 7 8 9 (1.0, 0.3, A)	9 1 2 3 4 5 6 7 8 9 (1.0, 0.0, A)	(40- 42)
K. Non-sustained nystagmus or dizziness during or immediately after provocative testing	4 2 1 _ 2 1 2 3 4 5 6 7 8 9 (2.0, 1.2, A)	5 1 _ 1 2 1 2 3 4 5 6 7 8 9 (1.0, 1.3, I)	7 _ 1 _ 1 1 2 3 4 5 6 7 8 9 (1.0, 0.7, A)	(43- 45)
L. History of unexplained syncope	_ 3 2 _ 3 _ 1 1 2 3 4 5 6 7 8 9 (3.0, 1.4, I)	4 2 _ _ 2 _ 1 1 2 3 4 5 6 7 8 9 (2.0, 1.7, I)	6 2 1 1 2 3 4 5 6 7 8 9 (1.0, 0.4, A)	(46- 48)
M. History of vague dizziness unexplained by other causes (anemia, orthostasis, electrolyte abnormalities, etc.)	_ _ 2 1 2 _ 3 1 1 2 3 4 5 6 7 8 9 (5.0, 1.6, I)	1 _ 1 2 1 _ 2 2 1 2 3 4 5 6 7 8 9 (5.0, 2.0, I)	4 _ 1 2 1 _ 1 1 2 3 4 5 6 7 8 9 (3.0, 1.8, I)	(49- 51)

Appropriateness scale: 1 = extremely inappropriate, 5 = uncertain, 9 = extremely appropriate.

REFERENCES

Arkuszewski, Z., "Involvement of the Cervical Spine in Back Pain, *Manual Medicine,* Vol. 2, 1986; pp. 126–128.

Beal, M. C., J. Vorro, and W. L. Johnston, "Chronic Cervical Dysfunction: Correlation of Myoelectric Findings with Clinical Progress," *Journal of the American Osteopathic Association,* Vol. 89, 1989, pp. 891–900.

Bergmann, T., and L. Porter, "Posterior Cervical Syndrome of Barre-Lieou," *Journal of Chiropractic Education,* Vol. 1, 1987, pp. 5–7.

Boline, P., and J. Meyer, "Chiropractic Management of Mechanical Cervical Spine Syndrome and Concomitant Myofascial Pain Syndrome: A Case Study," *Chiropractic Technique,* Vol. 2, 1990, pp. 176–181.

Boline, P. D., K. Kassak, C. Nelson, G. Bronfort, and A. Anderson, "Spinal Manipulation vs. Amitriptyline for the Treatment of Chronic Tension-type Headaches: A Randomized Clinical Trial." Submitted for publication, 1994.

Bonci, A., and C. Ratliff, "Strength Modulation of the Biceps Brachii Muscles Immediately Following a Single Manipulation of the C4/5 Intervertebral Motor Unit in Healthy Subjects: Preliminary Report," *American Journal of Chiropractic Medicine,* Vol. 3, 1990, pp. 14–18.

Bonebrake, A., J. Fernandez, J. Dahalan, and R. Marley, "A Treatment for Carpal Tunnel Syndrome: Results of a Follow-up Study," *Journal of Manipulative Physiological Therapeutics,* Vol. 16, 1993, pp. 125-139.

Bonebrake, A., J. Fernandez, R. Marley, J. Dahalan, and K. Kilmer, "A Treatment for Carpal Tunnel Syndrome: Evaluation of Objective and Subjective Measures," *Journal of Manipulative Physiological Therapeutics,* Vol. 13, 1990, pp. 507–520.

Brodin, H., "Cervical Pain and Mobilization," *Manual Medicine,* Vol. 2, 1985, pp. 18-22.

Burns, R., "The Cervical Spine in Manipulative Medicine," *Practitioner,* Vol. 222, 1979, pp. 803-806.

Carette, S., S. Marcoux, R. Truchon, C. Grondin, J. Gagnon, Y. Allard et al. "A Controlled Trial of Corticosteroid Injections into Facet Joints for Chronic Low Back Pain," *The New England Journal of Medicine*, Vol. 325, 1991, pp. 1002–1007.

Carlsson, J., A. Fahlcrantz, and L. Augustinsson, "Muscle Tenderness in Tension Headache Treated with Acupuncture or Physiotherapy," *Cephalalgia*, Vol. 10, 1990, pp. 131–141.

Cassidy, J. D., A. A. Lopes, and K. Yong-Hing, "The Immediate Effect of Manipulation Versus Mobilization on Pain and Range of Motion in the Cervical Spine: A Randomized Controlled Trial," *Journal of Manipulative Physiological Therapeutics*, Vol. 15, 1992a, pp. 570–575.

Cassidy, J. D., J. A. Quon, L. J. LaFrance, and K. Yong-Hing, "The Effect of Manipulation on Pain and Range of Motion in the Cervical Spine: A Pilot Study," *Journal of Manipulative Physiological Therapeutics*, Vol. 15, 1992b, pp. 495–500.

Christian, G. F., G. J. Stanton, D. Sissons, H. Y. How, J. Jamison, B. Alder, M. Fullerton, and J. W. Funder, "Immunoreactive ACTH, Beta-Endorphin, and Cortisol Levels in Plasma Following Spinal Manipulative Therapy," *Spine*, Vol. 13, 1988, pp. 1411–1417.

Detsky, A. S., C. D. Naylor, K. O'Rourke, A. J. McGreer, and K. A. L'Abbe, "Incorporating Variations in the Quality of Individual Randomized Trials into Meta-Analysis," *Journal of Clinical Epidemiology*, Vol. 45, No. 3, 1992, pp. 255–265.

Deyo, R. A., "Measuring the Functional Status of Patients with Low Back Pain," *Archives of Physical Medicine and Rehabilitation*, Vol. 69, 1988, pp. 1044–1053.

Dontigny, R. L., "Inhibition of Nausea and Headaches," *Physical Therapy*, Vol. 54, 1974, pp. 864–865.

Droz, J., and F. Crot, "Occipital Headaches," *Annals of the Swiss Chiropractors' Association*, Vol. 8, 1985, pp. 127–135.

Duff, B., "Documented Chiropractic Results on a Case Diagnosed as Myoclonic Seizures," *Chiropractic: The Journal of Chiropractic Research, Study and Clinical Investigation*, Vol. 8, 1992, pp. 56–57.

Fitz-Ritson, D. "Assessment of Cervicogenic Vertigo," *Journal of Manipulative Physiological Therapeutics*, Vol. 14, 1991, pp. 193–198.

Fitzgerald, R.T.D., "Observations on Trigger Points, Fibromyalgia, Recurrent Headache and the Cervical Syndrome," *Journal of Manual Medicine*, Vol. 6, 1991, pp. 124–129.

Glick, D. "Conservative Chiropractic Care of Cervicobrachalgia," *Chiropractic Research Journal*, Vol. 1, 1989, pp. 49–52.

Goodman, R., and J. Mosby, "Cessation of a Seizure Disorder: Correction of the Atlas Subluxation Complex," *Chiropractic: The Journal of Chiropractic Research, Study and Clinical Investigation*, Vol. 6, 1990, pp. 43–46.

Gorman, R. F., "Automated Static Perimetry in Chiropractic," *Journal of Manipulative Physiological Therapeutics*, Vol. 16, 1993, pp. 481–487.

Graff-Radford, S. B., J. L. Reeves, and B. Jaeger. "Management of Chronic Head and Neck Pain: Effectiveness of Altering Factors Perpetuating Myofascial Pain," *Headache*, Vol. 27, 1987, pp. 186–190.

Greenly, L., and T. Bergmann, "The Teres Syndrome," *Chiropractic Technique*, Vol. 2, 1990, pp. 56–58.

Grice, A., "Scalenus Anticus Syndrome Diagnosis and Chiropractic Adjustive Procedure," *Journal of the Canadian Chiropractors' Association*, Vol. 21, 1977, pp. 15–19.

Hammond, B., "Torticollis," *European Journal of Chiropractic*, Vol. 31, 1983, pp. 162–165.

Heilig, D., "Osteopathic Manipulative Medicine in Thoracic Outlet Syndrome," *Osteopathic Annals*, Vol. 3, 1975, pp. 19–32.

Hobbs, D., and S. Rasmussen, "Chronic Otitis Media: A Case Report," *Journal of Chiropractic*, Vol. 28, 1991, pp. 67-68.

Hoiriis, K., "Case Report: Management of Post-surgical Chronic Low Back Pain with Upper Cervical Adjustment," *Chiropractic Research Journal*, Vol. 1, 1989, pp. 37–42.

Howe, D. H., R. G. Newcombe, and M. T. Wade, "Manipulation of the Cervical Spine—A Pilot Study," *Journal of the Royal College of General Practice*, Vol. 33, 1983, pp. 564–579.

Hoyt, W., F. Shaffer, D. Bard, J. Benesler, G. Blankenhorn, J. Gray, W. Hartman, and L. Hughes, "Osteopathic Manipulation in the Treatment of Muscle-Contraction Headache," *Journal of the American Osteopathic Association*, Vol. 78, 1979, pp. 322–325.

Hruby, R., "The Total Body Approach to the Osteopathic Management of Temporomandibular Joint Dysfunction," *Journal of the American Osteopathic Association*, Vol. 85, 1985, pp. 502–510.

Hviid, H., "The Influence of the Chiropractic Treatment on the Rotary Mobility of the Cervical Spine—A Kinesiometric and Statistical Study," *Annals of the Swiss Chiropractors' Association*, Vol. 5, 1971, pp. 31–44.

Ingesson, E., E. Ribbe, and L. Norgren, "Thoracic Outlet Syndrome—Evaluation of a Physiotherapeutical Method," *Manual Medicine*, Vol. 2, 1986, pp. 86–88.

Jensen, O. K., F. F. Nielsen, and L. Vosmar, "An Open Study Comparing Manual Therapy with the Use of Cold Packs in the Treatment of Post-Traumatic Headache," *Cephalalgia*, Vol. 10, 1990, pp. 241–250.

Jirout, J., "The Effect of Mobilization of the Segmental Blockade on the Sagittal Component of the Reaction on Lateroflexion of the Cervical Spine, *Neuroradiology*, Vol. 3, 1972, pp. 210–215.

Jirout., J., "Comments Regarding the Diagnosis and Treatment of Dysfunctions in the C2-C3 Segment," *Manual Medicine*, Vol. 2, 1985, pp. 16–17.

Kettle, D., "The Effects of Manipulative Physiotherapy on Chronic Cervical Dysfunction," *Physiotherapy Theory and Practice*, Vol. 7, 1991, pp. 23–31.

Klougart, N., N. Nilsson, and J. Jacobsen, "Infantile Colic Treated by Chiropractors: A Prospective Study of 316 Cases," *Journal of Manipulative Physiological Therapeutics*, Vol. 12, 1989, pp. 281–288.

Koes, B. W., W. I. J. Assendelft, G. J. M. G. van der Heijden, and L. M. Bouter, "Spinal Manipulation and Mobilization for Back and Neck Pain: A Blinded Review," *British Medical Journal*, Vol. 303, 1991, pp. 1298–1303.

Koes, B. W., L. M. Bouter, H. van Mameren, A. H. Essers, G. J. Verstegen, D. M. Hofhuizen, J. P. Houben, and P. G. Knipschild, "A Randomized Clinical Trial of Manual Therapy and Physiotherapy for Persistent Back and Neck Complaints: Subgroup Analysis and Relationship Between Outcome Measures," *Journal of Manipulative Physiological Therapeutics*, Vol. 16, 1993, pp. 211–219.

Koes, B. W., L. M. Bouter, H. van Mameren, A. H. Essers, G. J. Verstegen, D. M. Hofhuizen, J. P. Houben, and P. G. Knipschild, "A Blinded Randomized Clinical Trial of Manual Therapy and Physiotherapy for Chronic Back and Neck Complaints: Physical Outcome Measures," *Journal of Manipulative Physiological Therapeutics*, Vol. 15, 1992a, pp. 16–23.

Koes, B. W., L. M. Bouter, H. van Mameren, A. H. Essers, G. J. Verstegen, D. M. Hofhuizen, J. P. Houben, and P. G. Knipschild, "Randomized Clinical Trial of Manipulative Therapy and Physiotherapy for Persistent Back and Neck Complaints: Results of One Year Follow Up," *British Medical Journal*, Vol. 304, 1992b, pp. 601–605.

Koes, B. W., L. M. Bouter, A. H. M. van Mameren, and A. H. Essers, "The Effectiveness of Manual Therapy, Physiotherapy, and Treatment by the General Practitioner for Monspecific Back and Neck Complaints: A Randomized Clinical Trial," *Spine*, Vol. 17, 1992c, pp. 28–35.

Kruse R., and D. Brodd, "Relief of Tension Headaches: A Case Study Using Chiropractic Manipulation and Acupuncture," *Journal of Chiropractic*, Vol. 28, 1991, pp. 57–59.

Leach, R., "An Evaluation of the Effect of Chiropractic Manipulative Therapy on Hypolordosis of the Cervical Spine," *Journal of Manipulative Physiological Therapeutics*, Vol. 6, 1983, pp. 17–24.

Lehman, J. J., "Manual Therapy in Upper Cervical Spinal Dysfunction," *Physiotherapy Journal of Canada*, Vol. 30, 1978, pp. 302–304.

Lewit, K. "Pain Arising in the Posterior Arch of the Atlas," *European Neurology*, Vol. 16, 1977, pp. 263–269.

Livingston, M., "Spinal Manipulation: A One-Year Follow-up Study," *Canadian Family Physician*, Vol. 15, 1969, pp. 35–39.

Livingston, M. C., "Spinal Manipulation in Medical Practice: A Century of Ignorance," *The Medical Journal of Australia*, Vol. 28, September 1968, pp. 552–555.

Lowden, T. A., J. C. J. Keating, and W. C. Meeker, "A Multivariate Time-Series Descriptive Case Study of Chiropractic Care in the Treatment of Cervical Pain," *Journal of Manipulative Physiological Therapeutics*, Vol. 9, 1986, pp. 267–277.

Mannen, E., "The Use of Cervical Radiographic Overlays to Assess Response to Manipulation: A Case Report," *Journal of the Canadian Chiropractors' Association*, Vol. 24, 1980, pp. 108–110.

Mariano, K., M. McDougle, and G. Tanksley, "Double Crush Syndrome: Chiropractic Care of an Entrapment Neuropathy," *Journal of Manipulative Physiological Therapeutics*, Vol. 14, 1991, pp. 262–265.

McAlpine, J., "Subluxation Induced Cervical Myelopathy: A Pilot Study," *Chiropractic Research Journal*, Vol. 2, 1991, pp. 7–22.

McConekey, C., S. Patterson, M. Waddell, and R. Steffen, "Pre- and Post-Thermographic Evaluation of Chiropractic Adjusting: A Case Report," *Journal of Chiropractic*, Vol. 27, 1990, pp. 73–74.

McKinney, L. A., "Early Mobilisation and Outcome in Acute Sprains of the Neck," *British Medical Journal*, Vol. 299, 1989a, pp. 1006–1008.

McKinney, L.A., J. O. Dornan, and M. Ryan, "The Role of Physiotherapy in the Management of Acute Neck Sprains Following Road-Traffic Accidents," *Archives of Emergency Medicine*, Vol. 6, 1989b, pp. 27–33.

McKnight, M. E., and K. F. DeBoer, "Preliminary Study of Blood Pressure Changes in Normotensive Subjects Undergoing Chiropractic Care," *Journal of Manipulative Physiological Therapeutics*, Vol. 11, 1988, pp. 261–266.

Mealy, K., H. Brennan, and G. C. Fenelon, "Early Mobilization of Acute Whiplash Injuries," *British Medical Journal (Clinical Research Edition)*, Vol. 292, 1986, pp. 656–657.

Mennell, J. M., "The Validation of the Diagnosis 'Joint Dysfunction' in the Synovial Joints of the Cervical Spine," *Journal of Manipulative Physiological Therapeutics*, Vol. 13, 1990, pp. 7–12.

Mierau, D., and J. Cassidy, "Degenerative Spondylolisthesis in the Cervical Spine: A Report of a Case," *Journal of the Canadian Chiropractors' Association*, Vol. 28, 1984, pp. 368–370.

Miller B., J. Maxwell, and K. DeBoer, "Chiropractic Treatment of Tension Headache: A Case Study," *Journal of Chiropractic*, Vol. 21, 1984, pp. 62–66.

Nansel, D., R. Jansen, E. Cremata, M. S. Dhami, and D. Holley, "Effects of Cervical Adjustments on Lateral-Flexion Passive End-Range Asymmetry and on Blood Pressure, Heart Rate and Plasma Catecholamine Levels," *Journal of Manipulative Physiological Therapeutics*, Vol. 14, 1991, pp. 450–456.

Nansel, D., A. Peneff, E. Cremata, and J. Carlson, "Time Course Considerations for the Effects of Unilateral Lower Cervical Adjustments with Respect to the Amelioration of Cervical Lateral-Flexion Passive End-Range Asymmetry," *Journal of Manipulative Physiological Therapeutics*," Vol. 13, 1990, pp. 297–304.

Nansel, D. D., E. Cremata, J. Carlson, and M. Szlazak, "Effect of Unilateral Spinal Adjustments on Goniometrically-Assessed Cervical Lateral-Flexion End-Range Asymmetries in Otherwise Asymptomatic Subjects," *Journal of Manipulative Physiological Therapeutics*, Vol. 12, 1989, pp. 419–427.

Nansel, D. D., A. Peneff, and J. Quitoriano, "Effectiveness of Upper Versus Lower Cervical Adjustments with Respect to the Amelioration of Passive Rotational Versus Lateral-Flexion End-Range Asymmetries in Otherwise Asymptomatic Subjects," *Journal of Manipulative Physiological Therapeutics*, Vol. 15, 1992, pp. 99–105.

Nansel, D.D., T. Waldorf, and R. Cooperstein, "Effect of Cervical Spinal Adjustments on Lumbar Paraspinal Muscle Tone: Evidence for Facilitation of Intersegmental Tonic Neck Reflexes," *Journal of Manipulative Physiological Therapeutics*, Vol. 16, 1993, pp. 91–95.

Nordemar, R., and C. Thorner, "Treatment of Acute Cervical Pain—A Comparative Group Study," *Pain*, Vol. 10, 1981, pp. 93–101.

Nykoliation, J., and J. Cassidy, "Manipulative Management of the Temporomandibular Joint Pain-Dysfunction Syndrome: A Report of Two Cases," *Journal of the Canadian Chiropractors' Association*, Vol. 28, 1984, pp. 257–262.

Parker, G. B., D. S. Pryor, and H. Tupling, "Why Does Migraine Improve During a Clinical Trial? Further Results from a Trial of Cervical Manipulation for Migraine," *Australian and New Zealand Journal of Medicine*, Vol. 10, 1980, pp. 192–198.

Parker, G. B., H. Tupling, and D. S. Pryor, "A Controlled Trial of Cervical Manipulation of Migraine," *Australian and New Zealand Journal of Medicine*, Vol. 8, 1978, pp. 589–593.

Passero, P., B. Wyman, J. Bell, S. Hirschey, and W. Schlosser, "Temporomandibular Joint Dysfunction Syndrome: A Clinical Report," *Physical Therapy*, Vol. 65, 1985, pp. 1203–1207.

Pedersen, P., "A Prospective Pilot Study of the Shape of Cervical Hypolordosis," *European Journal of Chiropractic*, Vol. 38, 1990, pp. 148–163.

Phillips, N., "Vertebral Subluxation and Otitis Media: A Case Study," *Journal of Chiropractic Research and Clinical Investigation*, Vol. 8, 1992, pp. 38–39.

Plaugher, G., E. E. Cremata, and R. B. Phillips, "A Retrospective Consecutive Case Analysis of Pretreatment and Comparative Static Radiological Parameters Following Chiropractic Adjustments," *Journal of Manipulative Physiological Therapeutics*, Vol. 13, 1990, pp. 498–506.

Rebechini, H., C Tasharski, and W. Heinze, "Electromyographic Analysis Following Chiropractic Manipulation of the Cervical Spine: A Model to Study Manipulation Induced Peripheral Muscle Changes," *Journal of Manipulative Physiological Therapeutics*, Vol. 4, 1981, pp. 61–63.

Robertson, A. M., "Manipulation in Cervical Syndromes," *Practitioner*, Vol. 200, 1968, pp. 396–402.

Robertson, J. A., "Manipulative Reduction of a Flexion Cervical Dysarthria: A Case Study," *Journal of Manipulative Physiological Therapeutics*, Vol. 1, 1978, pp. 113–116.

Robinson, S. S., K. F. Collins, and J. D. Grostic, "A Retrospective Study: Patients with Chronic Low Back Pain Managed with Specific Upper Cervical Adjustments," *Chiropractic Research Journal*, Vol. 2, 1993, pp. 10–16.

Rowe, L., and I. Steiman, "Anterolisthesis in the Cervical Spine—Spondylolysis," *Journal of Manipulative Physiological Therapeutics*, Vol. 10, 1987, pp. 11–20.

Rundcrantz, B. L., B. Johnsson, U. Moritz, and G. Roxendal, "Cervico-Brachial Disorders in Dentists: A Comparison Between Two Kinds of Physiotherapeutic Interventions," *Scandinavian Journal of Rehabilitative Medicine*, Vol. 23, 1991, pp. 11–17.

Sallstrom, J., and Z. Celegin, "Physiotherapy in Patients with Thoracic Outlet Syndrome," *VASA (Switzerland)*, Vol. 12, 1983, pp. 257–261.

Schultz, D., "Occipital Neuralgia," *Journal of the American Osteopathic Association*, Vol. 76, 1977, pp. 335–343.

Schutte, B., H. Teese, and J. Jamison, "Chiropractic Adjustments and Esophoria: A Retrospective Study and Theoretical Discussion," *Journal of the Australian Chiropractors' Association*, Vol. 19, 1989, pp. 126–128.

Shekelle, P. G., A. H. Adams, M. R. Chassin, E. L. Hurwitz, and R. H. Brook, "Spinal Manipulation for Low-Back Pain," *Annals of Internal Medicine*, Vol. 117, pp. 590–598.

Siciliano, M., T. Bernard, and N. Bentley, "Reduction of a Confirmed C5-C6 Disc Herniation Following Specific Chiropractic Spinal Manipulation: A Case Study," *Journal of Chiropractic Research and Clinical Investigation*, Vol. 8, 1992, pp. 17–23.

Sloop, P. R., D. S. Smith, E. Goldenberg, and C. Dore, "Manipulation for Chronic Neck Pain: A Double-Blind Controlled Study," *Spine*,Vol. 7, 1982, pp. 532–535.

Smith, K. F., "The Thoracic Outlet Syndrome: A Protocol of Treatment," *Journal of Orthopedic and Sports Physical Therapy*, Vol. 1, 1979, pp. 89–99.

Stodolny, J., and H. Chmielewski, "Manual Therapy in the Treatment of Patients with Cervical Migraine," *Journal of Manual Medicine*, Vol. 4, 1989, pp. 49–51.

Terrett, A. G. J., "Tinnitus, the Cervical Spine, and Spinal Manipulative Therapy," *Chiropractic Technique*, Vol. 1, 1989, pp. 41–45.

Trotta, N., "The Response of an Adult Tourette Patient to Life Upper Cervical Adjustments," *Chiropractic Research Journal*, Vol. 1, 1989, pp. 43–48.

Turk, Z., and O. Ratkolb, "Mobilization of the Cervical Spine in Chronic Headaches," *Manuelle Medizin*, Vol. 3, 1987, pp. 15–17.

Vaillancourt, P. J., and K. F. Collins, "Case Report: Management of Post-Surgical Low Back Syndrome with Upper Cervical Adjustment," *Chiropractic Research Journal*, Vol. 2, 1993, pp. 1–15.

Valente, R., "Chiropractic Therapy in Carpal Tunnel Syndrome: A Case Study," *Journal of Chiropractic*, Vol. 28, 1991, pp. 76–78.

van der Wendt, D. A. W. N., G. J. M. G. van der Heijden, R. J. P. M. Scholten, B. W. Koes, and L. M. Bouter, "The Efficacy of Non-Steroidal Anti-Inflammatory Drugs (NSAIDS) for Shoulder Complaints: A Systematic Review," *Journal of Clinical Epidemiology*, Vol. 48, No. 5, pp. 691–704.

Vernon, H., "The Role of Plethysmography in the Chiropractic Management of Costoclavicular Syndromes: Review of Principles and Case Report," *Journal of Manipulative Physiological Therapeutics*, Vol. 5, 1982a, pp. 17–20.

Vernon, H., "Chiropractic Manipulative Therapy in the Treatment of Headaches: A Retrospective and Prospective Study," *Journal of Manipulative Physiological Therapeutics*, Vol. 5, 1982b, pp. 109–112.

Vernon, H., "Pressure Pain Threshold Evaluation of the Effect of Spinal Manipulation on Chronic Neck Pain: A Single Case Study," *Journal of the Canadian Chiropractors' Association*, Vol. 32, 1988, pp. 191–194.

Vernon, H., "Spinal Manipulation and Headaches of Cervical Origin: A Review of Literature and Presentation of Cases," *Journal of Manual Medicine*, Vol. 6, 1991, pp. 73–79.

Vernon, H., M. Dhami, T. Howley, and R. Annett, "Spinal Manipulation and Beta-Endorphin: A Controlled Study of the Effect of a Spinal Manipulation on Plasma Beta-Endorphin," *Journal of Manipulative Physiological Therapeutics*, Vol. 9, 1986, pp. 115–123.

Vernon, H., and R. Gitelman, "Pressure Algometry and Tissue Compliance Measures in the Treatment of Chronic Headache by Spinal Manipulation: A Single Case Study," *Journal of the Canadian Chiropractors' Association*, Vol. 34, 1990, pp. 141–144.

Vernon, H. T., "Spinal Manipulation and Headaches of Cervical Origin," *Journal of Manipulative Physiological Therapeutics*, Vol. 12, 1989, pp. 455–468.

Vernon, H. T., P. Aker, S. Burns, S. Viljakaanen, and L. Short, "Pressure Pain Threshold Evaluation of the Effect of Spinal Manipulation in the Treatment of Chronic Neck Pain: A Pilot Study," *Journal of Manipulative Physiological Therapeutics*, Vol. 13, 1990, pp. 13–16.

Vernon, L. F., and D. C. Ehrenfeld, "Treatment of Temporomandibular Joint Syndrome for Relief of Cervical Spine Pain: Case Report," *Journal of Manipulative Physiological Therapeutics*, Vol. 5, 1982, pp. 79–81.

Wight, J., "Migraine: A Statistical Analysis of Chiropractic Treatment," *Journal of Chiropractic*, Vol. 15, 1978, pp. 63–67.

Wight, J. S., "Some Aspects of the Chiropractic Treatment for Migraine," *Bulletin of the European Chiropractic Union*, Vol. 28, 1980, pp. 15–24.

Wiles, M., "Observations on the Effects of Upper Cervical Manipulations on the Electrogastogram: A Preliminary Report," *Journal of Manipulative Physiological Therapeutics*, Vol. 3, 1980, pp. 226–229.

Wing, L. W., and W. Hargrave-Wilson, "Cervical Vertigo," *Australian and New Zealand Journal of Surgery*, Vol. 44, 1974, pp. 275–277.

Yeomans, S. G., "The Assessment of Cervical Intersegmental Mobility Before and After Spinal Manipulative Therapy," *Journal of Manipulative Physiological Therapeutics*, Vol. 15, 1992, pp. 106–114.

References on Treatment Complications

Beatty, R.A., "Dissecting Hematoma of the Internal Carotid Artery Following Chiropractic Cervical Manipulation," *Journal of Trauma*, Vol. 17, 1977, pp. 248–249.

Berciano, J., F. Coria, G. P. Anzola, and G. B. Frisoni, "Occipitoatlantal Instability: A Hemodynamic Cause of Vertebrobasilar Ischemia After Neck Motion," *Stroke*, Vol. 23, 1992, p. 921.

Blaine, E., "Manipulative (Chiropractic) Dislocations of the Atlas," *JAMA—Journal of the American Medical Association*, Vol. 85, 1925, pp. 1356–1359.

Braun, I.F., R. S. Pinto,, G. J. De Filipp, A. Lieberman, P. Pasternack and R. D. Zimmerman, "Brain Stem Infarction Due to Chiropractic Manipulation of the Cervical Spine," *Southern Medical Journal*, Vol. 76, 1983, pp. 1199–1201, 1507–1510.

Brownson, R. J., W. K. Zollinger, T. Madeira, and D. Fell, "Sudden Sensorineural Hearing Loss Following Manipulation of the Cervical Spine," *Laryngoscope*, Vol. 96, 1986, pp. 166–170.

Carmody, E., P. Buckley, and M. Hutchinson, "Basilar Artery Occlusion Following Chiropractic Cervical Manipulation," *Irish Medical Journal (Ireland)*, Vol. 80, 1987, pp. 259–260.

Cellerier, P., and A. Georget, "Dissection of Vertebral Arteries After Cervical Spine Manipulation," *Journal of Radiology*, Vol. 65, 1984, pp. 191–196.

Cervical Spine Research Society Editorial Committee, *The Cervical Spine*, 2nd edition, Philadelphia: J.B. Lippincott Company, 1989.

Cook, J. W., and J. K. Sanstead, "Wallenberg's Syndrome Following Self-Induced Manipulation," *Neurology*, Vol. 41, 1991, pp. 1695–1696.

Daneshmend, T., R. Hewer, and J. Bradshaw, "Acute Brain Stem Stroke During Neck Manipulation," *British Medical Journal*, Vol. 288, 1984, p. 189.

Davidson, K. C., E. C. Weiford, and G. D. Dixon, "Traumatic Vertebral Artery Pseudoaneurysm Following Chiropractic Manipulation," *Radiology*, Vol. 115, 1975, pp. 651–652.

Dunne, J. W., G. N. Conacher, M. Khangure, and C. G. Harper, "Dissecting Aneurysms of the Vertebral Arteries Following Cervical Manipulation: A Case Report," *Journal of Neurology, Neurosurgery and Psychiatry*, Vol. 50, 1987, pp. 349–353.

Dvorak, J., "Inappropriate Indications and Contraindications for Manual Therapy," *Manual Medicine*, Vol. 6, 1991, pp. 85–88.

Dvorak, J., H. Baumgartner, L. Burn, J. Dalgaard, E. Enevoldsen, J. Fossgreen, P. Greenman, and V. Janda, "Consensus and Recommendations as to the Side-Effects and Complications of Manual Therapy of the Cervical Spine," *Manual Medicine*, Vol. 6, 1991, pp. 117–118.

Dvorak, J., and F. Orelli, "How Dangerous Is Manipulation of the Cervical Spine? Case Report and Results of an Inquiry," *Manuelle Medizin*, Vol. 20, 1982, pp. 44–48.

Dvorak, J., and F. Orelli, "How Dangerous Is Manipulation to the Cervical Spine? Case Report and Results of a Survey," *Manual Medicine*, Vol. 2, 1985, pp. 1–4.

Easton, J. D., and D.G. Sherman, "Cervical Manipulation and Stroke," *Stroke*, Vol. 8, 1977, pp. 594–597.

Fast, A., D. F. Zinicola, and E. L. Marin, "Vertebral Artery Damage Complicating Cervical Manipulation," *Spine*, Vol. 12, 1987, pp. 840–842.

Ford, F. R., and D. Clark, "Thrombosis of the Basilar Artery with Softenings in the Cerebellum and Brain Due to Manipulation of the Neck," *Bulletin of The Johns Hopkins Hospital*, Vol. 98, 1956, pp. 37–42.

Frisoni, G. B., and G. P. Anzola, "Vertebrobasilar Ischemia After Neck Motion," *Stroke*, Vol. 22, 1991, pp. 1452–1460.

Fritz, V. U., A. Maloon, and P. Tuch, "Neck Manipulation Causing Stroke. Case Reports," *South African Medical Journal*, Vol. 66, 1984, pp. 844–846.

Frumkin, L. R., and R. W. Baloh, "Wallenberg's Syndrome Following Neck Manipulation," *Neurology*, Vol. 40, 1990, pp. 611–615.

Gabriel, S. E., L. Jaakkimainen, and C. Bombardier, "Risk for Serious Gastrointestinal Complications Related to Use of Nonsteroidal Anti-Inflammatory Drugs: A Meta-Analysis," *Annals of Internal Medicine*, Vol. 115, 1991, pp. 787–796.

Gittinger, J. W., "Occipital Infarction Following Chiropractic Cervical Manipulation," *Journal of Clinical Neuroophthalmology*, Vol. 6, 1986, pp. 11–13.

Goodbody, R. A., "Proceedings: Fatal Post-Traumatic Vertebro-Basilar Ischemia," *Journal of Clinical Pathology*, Vol. 29, 1976, pp. 86–87.

Gorman, R. F., "Cardiac Arrest After Cervical Spine Mobilization," *Medical Journal of Australia*, Vol. 2, 1978, pp. 169–170.

Gray, J., S. J. Phillips, and W. J. Maloney, "Vertebral Artery Dissection Following Cervical Chiropractic Manipulation," *NS Medical Journal*, Vol. 68, 1989, pp. 30–32.

Grayson, M. F., "Horner's Syndrome After Manipulation of the Neck," *British Medical Journal (Clin Res Ed)*, Vol. 295, 1987, pp. 1381–1382.

Green, D., and R. Joynt, "Vascular Accidents to the Brain Stem Associated with Neck Manipulation," *JAMA—Journal of the American Medical Association*, Vol. 170, 1959, pp. 522–524.

Gutmann, G., "Injuries to the Vertebral Artery Caused by Manual Therapy," *Manuelle Medizin*, Vol. 21, 1983, pp. 2–14.

Hamann, G. F., S. Felber, and K. Schimrigk, "Cervicocephalic Artery Dissections and Chiropractic Manipulations," *Lancet*, Vol. 342, 1993, p. 114.

Heffner, J. E., "Diaphragmatic Paralysis Following Chiropractic Manipulation of the Cervical Spine," *Archives of Internal Medicine*, Vol. 145, 1985, pp. 562–564.

Hinse, P., A. Thie, amd L. Lachenmayer, "Dissection of the Extracranial Vertebral Artery: Report of Four Cases and Review of the Literature," *Journal of Neurological and Neurosurgical Psychiatry*, Vol. 54, 1991, pp. 863–869.

Horn, S. W., "The 'Locked-In' Syndrome Following Chiropractic Manipulation of the Cervical Spine," *Annals of Emergency Medicine*, Vol. 12, 1983, pp. 648–650.

Jaskoviac, P., "Complications Arising from Manipulation of the Cervical Spine," *Journal of Manipulative Physiological Therapeutics*, Vol. 3, 1980, pp. 213–220.

Jentzen, J. M., J. Amatuzio, and G. F. Peterson, "Complications of Cervical Manipulation: A Case Report of Fatal Brainstem Infarct with Review of the Mechanisms and Predisposing Factors," *Journal of Forensic Science*, Vol. 32, 1987, pp. 1089–1094.

Kewalramani, L. S., D. L. Kewalramani, M. Krebs, and A. Saleem, "Myelopathy Following Cervical Spine Manipulation," *American Journal of Physical Medicine*, Vol. 61, 1982, pp. 165–175.

Krueger, B. R., and H. Okazaki, "Vertebral-Basilar Distribution Infarction Following Chiropractic Cervical Manipulation," *Mayo Clinic Proceedings*, Vol. 55, 1980, pp. 322–332.

Kunkle, E. C., Muller, J. C., and G. L. Odom, "Traumatic Brain Stem Thrombosis: Report of a Case and Analysis of the Mechanism of Injury," *Annals of Internal Medicine*, Vol. 36, 1952, pp. 1329–1335.

Ladermann, J., "Cerebrovascular Accidents Related to Chiropractic Care: Further Considerations," *European Journal of Chiropractic*, Vol. 38, 1990, pp. 63–68.

Lennington, B. R., D. W. Laster, D. M. Moody, and M. R. Ball, "Traumatic Pseudoaneurysm of Ascending Cervical Artery in Neurofibromatosis: Complication of Chiropractic Manipulation," *American Journal of Neuroradiology*, Vol. 1, 1980, pp. 269–270.

Lewis, M., and D. Grundy, "Vertebral Osteomyelitis Following Manipulation of Spondylitic Necks—A Possible Risk," *Paraplegia*, Vol. 30, 1992, pp. 788–790.

Lindy, D., "Patient Collapse Following Cervical Manipulation: A Case Report," *British Osteopathic Journal*, Vol. 16, 1984, pp. 84–85.

Lyness, S., and A. Wagman, "Neurological Deficit Following Cervical Manipulation," *Surgical Neurology*, Vol. 2, 1974, pp. 121–124.

Martienssen, J., and N. Nilsson, "Cerebrovascular Accidents Following Upper Cervical Manipulation: The Upper Cervical Manipulation," *American Journal of Chiropractic Medicine*, Vol. 29, 1989, pp. 160–163.

Mas, J. L., M. G. Bousser, P. J. Touboul, P. Hinse, and A. Thie, "Extracranial Vertebral Artery Dissection," *Journal of Neurological and Neurosurgical Psychiatry*, Vol. 55, 1992, pp. 979–980.

Mas, J. L., D. Henin, M. G. Bousser, F. Chain, and J. J. Hauw, "Dissecting Aneurysm of the Vertebral Artery and Cervical Manipulation: A Case Report with Autopsy," *Neurology*, Vol. 39, 1989, pp. 512–515.

Medical Economics Data, *Physicians' Desk Reference*, 47th edition, Montvale, N.J.: Medical Economics Company Inc., 1993.

Mehalic, T., and S. M. Farhat, "Vertebral Artery Injury from Chiropractic Manipulation of the Neck," *Surgical Neurology*, Vol. 2, 1974, pp. 125–129.

Miller, R. G., and R. Burton, "Stroke Following Chiropractic Manipulation of the Spine," *JAMA—Journal of the American Medical Association*, Vol. 229, 1974, pp. 189–190.

Mueller, S., and A. L. Sahs, "Brain Stem Dysfunction Related to Cervical Manipulation: Report of Three Cases," *Neurology*, Vol. 26, 1976, pp. 547–550.

Nyberg-Hansen, R., A. C. Loken, and O. Tenstad, "Brainstem Lesion with Coma for Five Years Following Manipulation of the Cervical Spine," *Journal of Neurology*, Vol. 218, 1978, pp. 97–105.

Pandit, A., "An Unusual Cause of Bilateral Diaphragmatic Paralysis," *Thorax*, Vol. 47, 1992, p. 201.

Parkin, P. J., W. E. Wallis, and J. L. Wilson, "Vertebral Artery Occlusion Following Manipulation of the Neck," *New Zealand Medical Journal*, Vol. 88, 1978, pp. 441–443.

Patijn, J., "Complications in Manual Medicine: A Review of the Literature," *Journal of Manual Medicine*, Vol. 6, 1991, pp. 89–92.

Povlsen, U. J., L. Kjaer, and P. Arlien-Soborg, "Locked-in Syndrome Following Cervical Manipulation," *Acta Neurologica Scandinavica*, Vol. 76, 1987, pp. 486–488.

Powell, F. C., W. C. Hanigan, and W. C. Olivero, "A Risk/Benefit Analysis of Spinal Manipulation Therapy for Relief of Lumbar or Cervical Pain," *Neurosurgery*, Vol. 33, 1993, pp. 73–78.

Pratt-Thomas, H. R., and K. E. Berger, "Cerebellar and Spinal Injuries After Chiropractic Manipulation," *JAMA—Journal of the American Medical Association*, Vol. 133, 1947, pp. 600–603.

Putman, T. D., and Y. Wu, "Tracheal Rupture Following Cervical Manipulation: Late Complication Posttracheostomy," *Archives of Physical Medicine and Rehabilitation*, Vol. 67, 1986, pp. 48–50.

Raskind, R., and C. M. North, "Vertebral Artery Injuries Following Chiropractic Cervical Spine Manipulation—Case Reports," *Angiology*, Vol. 41, 1990, pp. 445–452.

Rinsky, L. A., G. G. Reynolds, R. M. Jameson, and R. D. Hamilton, "A Cervical Spinal Cord Injury Following Chiropractic Manipulation," *Paraplegia*, Vol. 13, 1976, pp. 223–227.

Rothrock, J. F., J. R. Hesselink, and T. M. Teacher, "Vertebral Artery Occlusion and Stroke from Cervical Self-Manipulation," *Neurology*, Vol. 41, 1991, pp. 1696–1697.

Schellhas, K. P., R. E. Latchaw, L. R. Wendling, and L. H. Gold, "Vertebrobasilar Injuries Following Cervical Manipulation," *JAMA—Journal of the American Medical Association*, Vol. 244, 1980, pp. 1450–1453.

Schmidley, J., and T. Koch, "The Noncerebrovascular Complications of Chiropractic Manipulation," *Neurology*, Vol. 34, 1984, pp. 684–685.

Schmitt, H., "Axis Fracture After Chiropractic Manipulation on Spondylosis Carcinomatosa," *Manuelle Medizin*, Vol. 20, 1982, pp. 123–125.

Schmitt, H. P., "Anatomical Structure of the Cervical Spine with Reference to the Pathology of Manipulation Complications," *Journal of Manual Medicine*, Vol. 6, 1991, pp. 93–101.

Schwarz, G., A. Spano, and J. Geiger, "Posterior Inferior Cerebellar Artery Syndrome of Wallenberg After Chiropractic Manipulation," *Archives of Internal Medicine*, Vol. 97, 1956, pp. 352–354.

Shafrir, Y., and B. A. Kaufman, "Quadriplegia After Chiropractic Manipulation in an Infant with Congenital Torticollis Caused by a Spinal Cord Astrocytoma," *Journal of Pediatrics*, Vol. 120, 1992, pp. 266–269.

Shekelle, P. G., and R. M. Brook, "A Community-Based Study of the Use of Chiropractic Services," *American Journal of Public Health*, Vol. 81, 1991, pp. 439–442.

Sherman, D. G., R. G. Hart, and J. D. Easton, "Abrupt Change in Head Position and Cerebral Infarction," *Stroke*, Vol. 12, 1981, pp. 2–6.

Sherman, M. R., J. E. Smialek, and W. E. Zane, "Pathogenesis of Vertebral Artery Occlusion Following Cervical Spine Manipulation," *Archives of Pathology and Laboratory Medicine*, Vol. 111, 1987, pp. 851–853.

Simmons, K. C., Y. S. Soo, G. Walker, and P. Harvey, "Trauma to the Vertebral Artery Related to Neck Manipulation," *Medical Journal of Australia*, Vol. 1, 1982, pp. 187–188.

Sinel, M., and D. Smith, "Thalamic Infarction Secondary to Cervical Manipulation," *Archives of Physical Medicine and Rehabilitation*, Vol. 74, 1993, pp. 543–546.

Smith, R., and M. Estridge, "Neurologic Complications of Head and Neck Manipulations: Report of Two Cases," *JAMA—Journal of the American Medical Association*, Vol. 182, 1962, pp. 528–531.

Stuart, P. J., T. Bernstein, L. E. Bertolucci, P. Uriell, and C. Swaffer, "A Case of Subdural Hematoma and Temporal Bone Fracture as Complications of Chiropractic Manipulation," *Journal of Emergency Medicine*, Vol. 7, 1989, pp. 615–617.

Sullivan, E., "Brain Stem Stroke Syndromes from Cervical Adjustments: Report on Five Cases," *Journal of Chiropractic Research and Clinical Investigation*, Vol. 8, 1992, pp. 12–16.

Terrett, A., "Importance and Interpretation of Tests Designed to Predict Susceptibility to Neurocirculatory Accidents," *Journal of the Australian Chiropractors' Association*, Vol. 13, 1983, pp. 29–34.

Terrett, A., "Vascular Accidents from Cervical Spine Manipulation: Report on 107 Cases," *Journal of the Australian Chiropractors' Association*, Vol. 17, 1987, pp. 15–24.

Terrett, A., "It Is More Important to Know When Not to Adjust," *Chiropractic Technique*, Vol. 1, 1990, pp. 1–9.

Terrett, A., and M. Webb, "Vertebrobasilar Accidents (VA) Following Cervical Spine Adjustment Manipulation," *Journal of the Australian Chiropractors' Association*, Vol. 12, 1982, pp. 24–27.

Tolge, C., V. Iyer, and J. McConnell, "Phrenic Nerve Palsy Accompanying Chiropractic Manipulation of the Neck," *Southern Medical Journal*, Vol. 86, 1993, pp. 688–690.

Weinstein, S. M., and R. C. Cantu, "Cerebral Stroke in a Semi-Pro Football Player: A Case Report," *Medicine and Science in Sports and Exercise*, Vol. 23, 1991, pp. 1119–1121.

Weintraub, M., "Dormant Foramen Magnum Meningioma 'activated' by Chiropractic Manipulation," *New York Journal of Medicine*, Vol. 83, 1983, pp. 1039–1040.

Zak, S., and R. Carmody, "Cerebellar Infarction from Chiropractic Neck Manipulation," *Arizona Medicine*, Vol. 41, 1984, pp. 333–337.

Zauel, D., and T. J. Carlow, "Internuclear Ophthalmoplegia Following Cervical Manipulation," *Annals of Neurology*, Vol. 1, 1977, p. 308.

Zimmerman, A. W., A. J. Kumar, N. Gadoth, and F. J. Hodges, "Traumatic Vertebrobasilar Occlusive Disease in Childhood," *Neurology*, Vol. 28, 1978, pp. 185–188.

Zupruk, G. M., Z. Mehta, and R. B. Morawetz, "Brown-Sequard Syndrome Associated with Posttraumatic Cervical Epidural Hematoma: Case Report and Review of the Literature," *Neurosurgery*, Vol. 25, 1989, pp. 278–280.